Essentials of Periodontics

Essentials of Periodontics

PHILIP M. HOAG, D.D.S., F.I.C.D., F.A.C.D.

Professor of Periodontics and Head,
Department of Periodontics, College of Dentistry,
University of Illinois at Chicago,
Chicago, Illinois

ELIZABETH A. PAWLAK, R.D.H., B.S., M.S. Ed.

Formerly Assistant Professor of Dental Hygiene,
William Rainey Harper College,
Palatine, Illinois

FOURTH EDITION

with **380** *illustrations*

original drawings by **Christo M. Popoff**

The C. V. Mosby Company

ST. LOUIS · BALTIMORE · PHILADELPHIA · TORONTO   1990

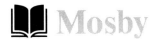

Editor: Robert W. Reinhardt
Assistant Editor: Melba Steube
Design: Rey Umali
Editing and production: Cracom Corp.

FOURTH EDITION

The C.V. Mosby Company
11830 Westline Industrial Drive, St. Louis, Missouri 63146

Library of Congress Cataloging in Publication Data

Hoag, Philip M.
    Essentials of periodontics/Philip M. Hoag, Elizabeth A. Pawlak;
original drawings by Christo M. Popoff.—4th ed.
      p. cm.
    Pawlak's name appears first on the 3rd ed.
    Includes bibliographies and index.
    ISBN 0-8016-2228-X
    1. Periodontics. I. Pawlak, Elizabeth A.   II. Title.
    [DNLM: 1. Periodontal Diseases.   WU 240 H678e]
RK361.H62 1990
617.6′32—dc19

C/D/D 9 8 7 6 5 4 3 2 1

Contributors

ARTHUR N. BAHN, A.B., M.A., Ph.D.

Professor and Head, Section of Microbiology, Department of Biomedical Sciences, School of Dental Medicine, Southern Illinois University of Edwardsville, Edwardsville, Illinois; Adjunct Professor of Oral Pathology, School of Dentistry, Medical University of South Carolina, Charleston, South Carolina

MARY M. LEE, R.D., Dr.P.H.

Nutrition Program Consultant, Nutrition and Dietary Services Branch, Division of Health Services, North Carolina Department of Human Resources, University of North Carolina at Chapel Hill, Chapel Hill, North Carolina

To
OUR STUDENTS

Preface

The prevention and treatment of diseases affecting the periodontium are becoming increasingly important to the public and the dental profession. National surveys indicate that more people are keeping their teeth longer and that there is an increase in the middle and older age groups who traditionally need and seek periodontal treatment. In addition, the amount and quality of public awareness literature in regard to periodontics has increased dramatically. This increase means that the demands placed on the dental team for current, factual information concerning the causes and treatment of periodontal diseases will continue to grow in the years ahead.

Our purpose in the preparation of this book is to provide a concise and selective coverage of the basic principles and techniques involved in periodontics. A book of this nature cannot provide all the information on such a growing and detailed field; therefore we strongly recommend that readers use the suggested reading lists provided at the end of each chapter to further expand and stimulate their learning.

The book is written to provide for ease of learning and reference. Each periodontal disease is discussed on the basis of 10 key factors and presented in a modified outline form: (1) definition, (2) clinical characteristics, (3) radiographic changes, (4) histopathology and pathogenesis, (5) etiology, (6) prognosis, (7) nutritional implications, (8) treatment, (9) patient education, and (10) preventive measures.

In this edition the clinical relevance of the information has been updated with new photographs, radiographs, and drawings. The text has been revised with major additions in the areas of periodontal microbiology and immunology, early onset periodontal diseases, adult learning as it applies to patient education and instruction, antimicrobial therapy, scaling and root planing, and periodontal surgery.

This book is written primarily for use by dental hygiene and dental assisting students. However, dental students as well as many experienced members of the dental health team who are involved in periodontics should find it of interest. Because of its concise nature it can be a valuable aid in continuing education programs as well as a reference in the dental office.

This is the fourth edition of *Essentials of Periodontics*. We thank you for your comments on the content, approach, and illustrations of the previous editions that enabled this revision to be modified to better meet the growing needs of the student, instructor, and practitioner. Again, we will appreciate additional comments. We trust that this book will be an enjoyable learning experience and will stimulate further study.

Philip M. Hoag
Elizabeth A. Pawlak

Contents

Essentials of Periodontics

CHAPTER 1
Periodontal Anatomy: Clinical and Histological Characteristics

Knowledge of the anatomy of the periodontal tissues and their associated structures is essential to understanding periodontal diseases and their treatment. This chapter describes the clinical and microscopic features of healthy periodontal tissues.

PERIODONTIUM

The tissues that surround and support the teeth are known as the *periodontium*. Anatomically the periodontal structures are described (Fig. 1-1) as the following:

1. Gingiva
2. Periodontal ligament
3. Alveolar bone
4. Cementum

GINGIVA

The gingiva is one of the soft tissues that line the oral cavity. Collectively all the soft tissues of the mouth are known as the oral mucosa. They are divided into three different types as follows:

1. *Masticatory mucosa* is tissue that is firmly attached to the underlying bone and covered with parakeratinized or keratinized epithelium. It is designed to withstand the frictional forces of food skirting over it during chewing and swallowing. The gingiva and the tissue covering the hard palate are examples of masticatory mucosa.
2. *Lining mucosa* is composed of oral tissues that are loosely attached to their underlying structures and covered with nonkeratinized epithelium. The oral tissues that make up this type are the mucosa covering the lips, cheeks, floor of the mouth, inferior surface of the tongue, soft palate, uvula, and alveolar mucosa.
3. *Specialized mucosa* covers the dorsal surface of the tongue and is adapted to accommodate for the sensation of taste.

The gingiva is the soft tissue adjacent to the cervical portions of the teeth. It is attached to the teeth and provides a covering for the coronal portion of the alveolar bone.

Types of gingiva

The gingiva can be divided into three contiguous areas (Figs. 1-2 to 1-4): (1) marginal (free or unattached), (2) attached (firmly attached to underlying tooth and bone), and (3) interdental (located between adjacent teeth).

Marginal gingiva

The marginal gingiva is the most coronally positioned portion of the gingiva. It is not attached to the tooth, and it creates the soft tissue wall of the *gingival sulcus* (the shallow space between the marginal gingiva and the tooth) (Fig. 1-4). In health the marginal gingiva is knife-edged in contour, firm in consistency, and smooth in texture. It extends apically to the *free gingival groove*, a shallow depression in the gingival surface approximately 1 mm

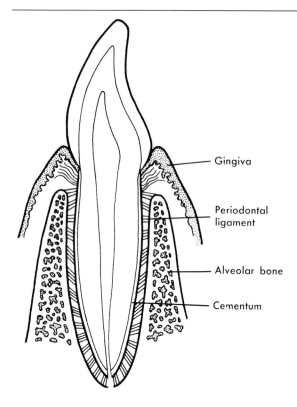

Gingiva

Periodontal ligament

Alveolar bone

Cementum

FIGURE 1-1. Faciolingual histological section illustrating the tissues comprising the periodontium.

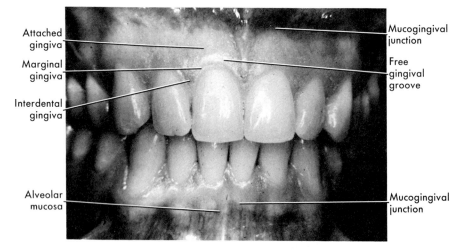

Attached gingiva

Marginal gingiva

Interdental gingiva

Alveolar mucosa

Mucogingival junction

Free gingival groove

Mucogingival junction

FIGURE 1-2. Healthy gingival tissues in a 21-year-old man. Note tapered contours, pointed interdental gingiva, free gingival groove, stippled texture, and mucogingival junction.

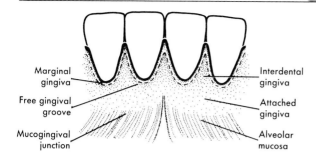

FIGURE 1-3. Divisions of the gingiva: marginal gingiva, attached gingiva, interdental gingiva, and the adjacent structures, mucogingival junction and alveolar mucosa.

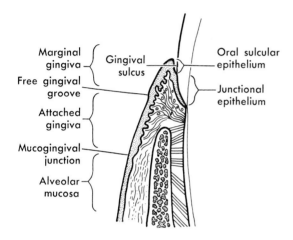

FIGURE 1-4. Faciolingual histological section of the periodontium on the facial surface of a tooth.

wide that corresponds to the most coronal aspect of the gingival attachment to the tooth. In some patients the free gingival groove is pronounced, while in others it is absent.

Attached gingiva

Just apical to the marginal gingiva and the free gingival groove is the attached gingiva. It is firmly bound to the underlying tooth and alveolar bone (Figs. 1-2 to 1-4). The attached gingiva is tapered in contour, stippled in texture, and firm in consistency. (Stippling refers to the irregular surface of the gingiva, which resembles the surface of an orange.) The attached gingiva varies in width from one area of the mouth to another and can range from less than 1 mm to 9 mm. The width depends principally on the teeth involved, their buccolingual position in the arch, and the location of frena or muscle attachments. In general the attached gingiva is widest on the incisor teeth, ranging from 3.5 to 4.5 mm in the maxilla and 3.3 to 3.9 mm in the mandible. The attached gingiva is narrower on the posterior teeth with the premolar areas being approximately 1.9 mm in the maxilla and 1.8 mm in the mandible (Fig. 1-2). It provides gingival tissue that can withstand the mechanical forces of toothbrushing and prevents movement of the marginal gingiva when tension is placed on the alveolar mucosa. In the past at least a minimal width of attached gingiva was considered necessary for gingival health, but recent studies have shown that gingival health and attachment levels can be maintained in the absence of attached gingiva. The attached gingiva is bound coronally by the free

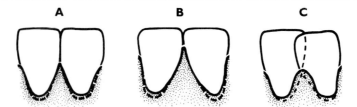

FIGURE 1-5. Effect of tooth contours and positions on the shape of the interdental gingiva. **A,** Flat tooth contours and broad interproximal contact areas cause short and narrow gingiva. **B,** Convex tooth contours and small contact areas create broad and high gingiva. **C,** Overlapping teeth make the interproximal space small, resulting in gingiva that bulge out of the confines of the space.

gingival groove and apically by the mucogingival junction. The latter demarks the beginning of the alveolar mucosa (Figs. 1-2 to 1-4), which is loosely attached to the underlying bone, smooth in surface texture, covered with a thin layer of nonkeratinized epithelium, and generally not as resistant to frictional contact as the attached gingiva.

Keratinized gingiva is covered with keratinized or parakeratinized stratified squamous epithelium. This includes the free or marginal gingiva as well as the attached gingiva and should be differentiated from the attached gingiva, which does not include the unattached tissues that form the soft tissue walls of the healthy sulcus or a pocket.

Interdental gingiva

The interdental gingiva is located in the interproximal space created by adjacent teeth in contact (Figs. 1-2 and 1-3). In the mesiodistal dimension the shape of the interdental gingiva, while generally triangular, depends on the proximal contours of the teeth creating the interproximal space. If the contours are flat with broad interproximal contacts, the gingiva will be narrow and short (Fig. 1-5, A). If the proximal contours are more convex with a small coronally positioned contact area, the interdental gingiva will be broad and high (Fig. 1-5, B). When teeth overlap, the interdental space is small or absent, resulting in bulbous gingiva (Fig. 1-5, C).

In the buccolingual dimension the interdental gingiva terminates coronally with separate buccal and lingual peaks of tissue joined by a depression known as the *gingival col* (Fig. 1-6, A).

If the gingival tissue has receded to the point that it no longer touches the interproximal contact areas or if diastemata are present, no col (Fig. 1-7) will be seen. The col is present only when the gingiva surrounds the gingival surface of the interproximal contact area (Fig. 1-6, B).

Gingival sulcus, sulcular epithelium, probing depth, and junctional epithelium

The gingival sulcus is the shallow space between the marginal gingiva and the tooth. Histologically the sulcus is lined with nonkeratinized (sulcular) epithelium and extends from the crest of the marginal gingiva to the most coronal level of the junctional epithelium (Figs. 1-4 and 1-8, A and C). The average depth is 1.8 mm with variations up to 0.6 mm. The healthy gingival sulcus depth as determined clinically with a periodontal probe (probing depth) is slightly deeper (2 to 3 mm) than the histologically measured depth because the probe often penetrates the delicate epithelial lining of the gingival sulcus. The junctional epithelium, which is located apical to the sulcular epithelium, is approximately 1 to 2 mm in length and attaches the gingiva to the tooth. It establishes the histological gingival attachment level and is

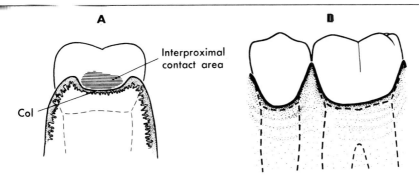

FIGURE 1-6. Shape of the interdental gingiva in the buccolingual dimension. **A,** Gingival col—the concave buccolingual contour of the interdental gingiva when it occupies the entire interproximal embrasure space. **B,** Appearance from the buccal aspect of the interdental gingiva that occupies the entire interproximal space and has a col as shown in **A.**

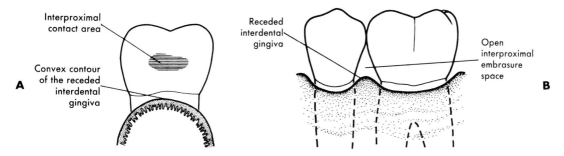

FIGURE 1-7. Shape of the interdental gingiva following gingival recession. **A,** Convex buccolingual contour of the interdental gingiva. **B,** Blunted appearance of the interdental gingiva from the buccal aspect.

formed by a uniting of the oral epithelium and the reduced enamel epithelium during tooth eruption.

Histology (Fig. 1-8)

An understanding of the clinical features of the periodontium is enhanced by a knowledge of the component tissues as seen microscopically.

Epithelium

The gingival tissues are made up of fibrous connective tissue covered by stratified squamous epithelium. The epithelium that covers the oral surface of the attached and marginal gingiva is either parakeratinized or kerati-

nized, while the sulcular epithelium and the junctional epithelium are nonkeratinized. The sulcular epithelium is thinner, which makes it easier for the products of dental plaque to penetrate into the connective tissue of the gingiva and stimulate inflammation and tissue destruction. The epithelium that covers the alveolar mucosa is thin and nonkeratinized.

The oral epithelium that is keratinized or parakeratinized is composed of four layers of cells (Fig. 1-8, *C*). The deepest cells are cuboidal in shape (basal cells) and form the *stratum basale*. The second layer of cells, called the *stratum spinosum*, is composed of polygonal cells. The next layer is composed of cells that are flattened in shape with prominent basophilic keratohyaline granules in the cytoplasm. This layer is known as the *stratum granulosum*. The most superficial layer, the *stratum corneum*, is a cornified layer that may be keratinized (no nuclei), parakeratinized (retained nuclei), or both. The epithelial cells are formed as basal cells and gradually change to the characteristics of each of the cell layers as they migrate toward the surface. This process is known as keratinization. The cells are ultimately sloughed from the keratinized surface layer. The cell turnover rate in experimental animals is about 10 to 12 days for the oral epithelium and 1 to 6 days for the junctional epithelium.

The epithelial cells are joined together by structures known as desmosomes, tight junctions, and intercellular ground substance. The basal cells are attached to the basement membrane by hemidesmosomes.

The junction between keratinized gingival oral epithelium and its underlying connective tissue is usually wavy in shape. The projections of epithelial cells into the connective tissue are known as *rete pegs*. The intervening projections of connective tissue are known as *connective tissue papillae* (Fig. 1-8, A). The alternating pattern of connective tissue papillae and epithelial rete pegs is thought to be related to the stippled (orange peel) surface texture of attached gingiva.

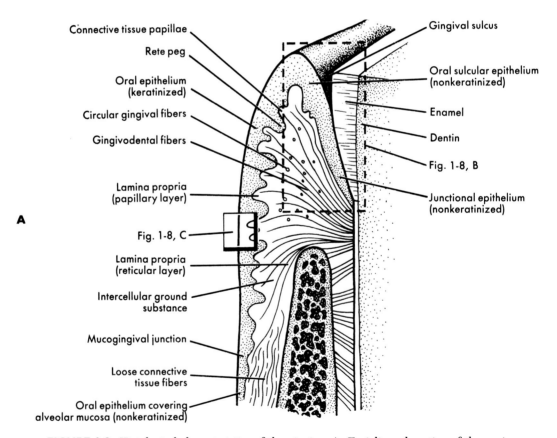

FIGURE 1-8. Histological characteristics of the gingiva. **A,** Faciolingual section of the periodontium.

The thickness of the gingival epithelium is maintained by a balance between new basal cell formation and the sloughing of older cells at the surface. The crevicular epithelium and the junctional epithelium are not as thick as the oral epithelium, are not keratinized, and in health have no rete pegs. The epithelium in these areas is composed principally of the stratum basale and the stratum spinosum.

The basal cells in the junctional epithelium are joined to the tooth by hemidesmosomes and a basal lamina. This attachment is similar to that between epithelium and fibrous connective tissue. The basal lamina is composed of a lamina densa adjacent to the tooth surface and a lamina lucida to which the hemidesmosomes of the epithelial cells are attached.

Connective tissue

The connective tissue of the gingiva is known as the lamina propria. It is divided into two layers: (1) the papillary layer, adjacent to the epithelium, and (2) the reticular layer, contiguous with the periosteum on the alveolar bone. The lamina propria consists primarily of the following (Fig. 1-8, A):

1. Collagen fibers
2. Intercellular ground substance
3. Cells
4. Blood vessels
5. Nerves

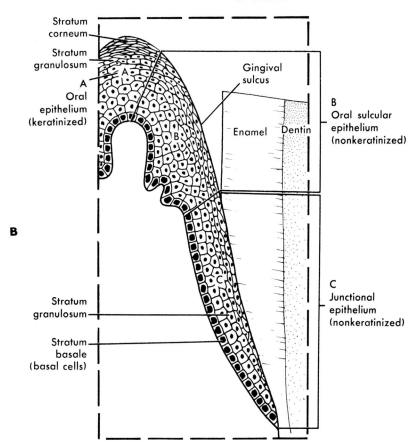

FIGURE 1-8, cont'd. B, Detail of the sulcular junctional epithelium areas.

Continued.

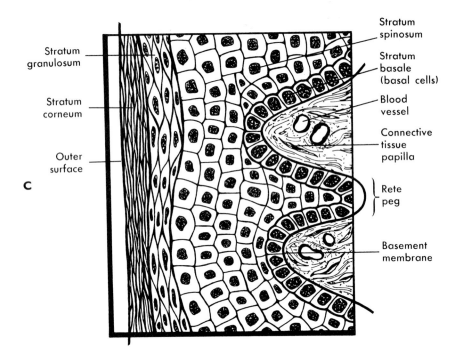

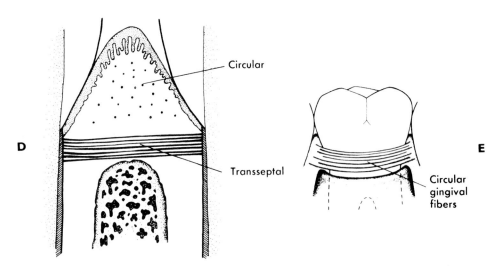

FIGURE 1-8, cont'd. **C,** Four layers (strata) of epithelial cells found in keratinized oral epithelium. **D,** Mesiodistal section of an interproximal area of the periodontium illustrating the transseptal and circular gingival fibers. **E,** Circular gingival fibers in the gingiva on the buccal aspect of a molar tooth.

The collagen fibers help to hold the marginal gingiva tightly against the tooth and provide a firm junction of the attached gingiva to the underlying tooth root and alveolar bone. The fibers are grouped into the following classification:

1. Gingivodental (Fig. 1-8, *A*)
2. Circular (Fig. 1-8, *A, D,* and *E*)
3. Transseptal (Fig. 1-8, *D*)

The gingivodental group runs from the root surface out into the gingiva, the circular group runs circumferentially around the tooth, and the transseptal group runs between adjacent teeth.

Collagen fibers are strong ropelike cords that bind and hold tissues together in functioning units. Their structure consists of three polypeptide chains wound together to form a basic collagen molecule. The molecules aggregate side by side to form collagen filaments, which in turn are accumulated to form the collagen fibril. The collagen fibers found in the gingival fibers are composed of many collagen fibrils held together by proteoglycans.

In contrast to the dense mass of firmly bound collagen fibers found in the gingiva, the connective tissue of the alveolar mucosa is composed of more loosely arranged collagen fibers interspersed with elastic and muscle fibers (Fig. 1-8, *A*). They are not firmly attached to the underlying bone, and therefore this tissue can be moved easily to adapt to the changing shapes and sizes of the muscles during function.

The viscous intercellular ground substance consists principally of mucopolysaccharides and glycoproteins. These substances help to regulate the distribution of water, electrolytes, and metabolites in the tissues.

Following are the most prominent cells found in the gingival connective tissue:

1. Plasma cells
2. Fibroblasts
3. Mast cells
4. Lymphocytes

Vascular supply

The blood supply to the periodontium is derived from the following branches of the superior and inferior alveolar arteries (Fig. 1-9):

1. *Supraperiosteal arteries* on the facial, lingual, and palatal surfaces of the alveolar bone
2. *Interdental arteries* located within the interproximal bone that exit at the crest of the interproximal alveolar processes to supply the gingiva
3. *Periodontal ligament arterioles*

The blood supply to the gingiva is profuse with multiple capillary loops extending throughout the lamina propria and into each connective tissue papilla. This profuse blood supply is why the color variations are so easily seen with the vascular changes of gingivitis.

The lymphatic drainage usually follows the blood supply, with the major portion of the lymph drainage from the gingiva going to the submandibular lymph nodes.

Nerves

The innervation of the gingiva is derived from the maxillary and mandibular branches of the trigeminal nerve. The buccal gingiva of the maxillary posterior teeth is supplied by the superior alveolar nerve, and the facial gingiva of the maxillary incisors and cuspids is supplied by the labial branch of the infraorbital nerve. The nasopalatine nerve supplies the palatal gingiva of the maxillary anterior teeth, and the anterior palatal nerve supplies the maxillary posterior teeth. The buccal gingiva of the mandibular molars and premolars is supplied by the long buccal nerve, while the facial gingiva of the anterior teeth is supplied by the mental nerve. The lingual gingiva of all the mandibular teeth is supplied by the lingual nerve.

Gingival fluid

The gingival (crevicular) fluid is continually secreted from the gingival connective tissues into the sulcus through the sulcular epithelial wall.

A

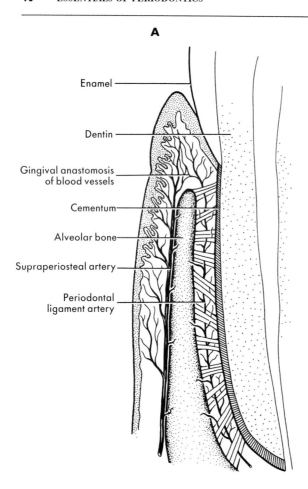

Enamel

Dentin

Gingival anastomosis
of blood vessels

Cementum

Alveolar bone

Supraperiosteal artery

Periodontal
ligament artery

FIGURE I-9. Blood supply to the periodontium. **A,** Supraperiosteal and periodontal ligament arteries on the facial or lingual surface of a tooth.

This fluid helps to mechanically clean the sulcus and in addition, possesses antimicrobial properties and antibodies that enhance the resistance of the gingiva to gingivitis. It also contains plasma proteins, which may improve the adhesion of the epithelium to the tooth. Secretion of crevicular fluid increases when the tissues are inflamed and when the patient is chewing. It also increases when a patient is pregnant or taking contraceptive medication. This increase is most likely related to the exaggerated inflammatory response to local irritants associated with these hormonal changes. The crevicular fluid is most commonly considered

to be an inflammatory exudate; however, small amounts are found in clinically healthy gingival sulci.

Clinical descriptive criteria
Gingival color

The color of healthy gingiva is uniformly coral pink from the attached gingiva through to the crest of the marginal gingiva (Fig. 1-2). However, considerable variation exists, depending on the amount of melanin in the tissues, the thickness of the epithelium, the degree of keratinization, and the vascularity of the connective tissue. Dark-skinned people often exhibit a

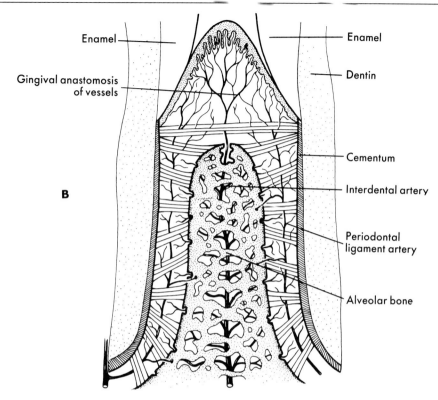

Enamel

Gingival anastomosis of vessels

B

Enamel

Dentin

Cementum

Interdental artery

Periodontal ligament artery

Alveolar bone

FIGURE I-9, cont'd. B, Mesiodistal section of an interproximal area of the periodontium illustrating the interdental and the periodontal ligament arteries.

dark blue or brown color. Red to bluish-red changes are often characteristic of gingival inflammation.

Gingival contour

The marginal and attached gingiva are usually tapered in contour, ending coronally in knife-edged margins. The interdental gingiva is generally pointed. However, the contours of the gingiva vary depending upon the shape of the teeth, the buccolingual position of the teeth in the arch, and the size of the interproximal embrasure space. In gingival disease the contours are often rounded and enlarged because of vascular stagnation and increased formation of collagen fibers.

Gingival consistency

In health the gingiva is usually resilient and firm because of the dense collagenous nature of the gingival connective tissue. In gingival disease the consistency may be soft and boggy, because of vascular stagnation and a decrease in the amount of gingival collagen fibers, or extremely firm, because of excessive formation of collagen (fibrosis).

Gingival surface texture

The surface texture of the gingiva is described as being stippled like an orange peel or smooth and shiny. The attached gingiva and the central portions of the interdental gingiva are stippled, and the marginal gingiva is smooth. The degree of stippling varies considerably among patients and in different parts of the same mouth. A reduction or lack of stippling is frequently seen in inflamed gingiva.

Gingival position

The level on the tooth at which the gingiva is attached is known as the gingival position. When teeth first erupt into the oral cavity the gingival attachments are close to the tips of the crowns; however, they generally shift to the areas of the cementoenamel junctions during the eruption and aging process. In periodontal disease the gingival position (attachment) is found on the root surface. The measurement of gingival attachment levels is made with a periodontal probe from the most coronal level of the junctional epithelium to a fixed reference point on the tooth (most commonly the cementoenamel junction.)

PERIODONTAL LIGAMENT

The periodontal ligament is the composite of tissues that surround the root of the tooth and serve as the attachment of the tooth to the alveolar bone. It consists primarily of bundles of continuous intermingling collagen fibers arranged into a network running from the tooth to the alveolar bone proper. These fibers are referred to as the *principal fibers of the periodontal ligament*. In teeth undergoing active eruption it has been suggested that the fiber bundles consist of three separate sections. One section is located toward the cementum, one toward the alveolar bone, and one area of splicing known as the intermediate plexus is located midway between the root and the bone. This plexus has not been identified in fully erupted human teeth. The average width of the periodontal ligament of an adult tooth in function is 0.18 mm. However, it has an hourglass shape, being widest in the coronal aspect, slightly narrower near the apex, and narrowest in the middle of the alveolus in the area of rotation.

The principal collagen fibers are arranged into the following four groups (Fig. 1-10):

1. Alveolar crestal fibers
2. Horizontal fibers
3. Oblique fibers
4. Apical fibers

The alveolar crestal fibers run from the tooth to the crest of the alveolar bone in an apical direction. The horizontal fibers are located just apical to the alveolar crestal fibers and run perpendicularly from the tooth to the alveolar bone. The oblique fibers, which comprise the largest group, run in a coronal direction from the tooth to the bone. The apical fibers radiate around the apex of the tooth to the adjacent bone.

The ends of the principal fibers are embedded in cementum on the tooth side and in the alveolar bone proper on the opposite side. The embedded portions of the principal fibers are known as *Sharpey's fibers* (Fig. 1-10).

Surrounding the collagen fibers is a looser type of connective tissue within which cells, blood, lymph vessels, and nerves are found.

The blood vessels found in the periodontal ligament are branches from three sources: the apical vessels that supply the teeth, the vessels in the interproximal alveolar bone, and the gingival vessels (Fig. 1-9).

Following are the principal cells found in the periodontal ligament:

1. Undifferentiated mesenchymal cells
2. Fibroblasts
3. Osteoblasts
4. Osteoclasts
5. Cementoblasts
6. Epithelial rests of Malassez

With the exception of the epithelial rests of Malassez, which are the remnants of the Hertwig root sheath, these cells are involved in the destruction and formation of the tissues of the periodontal ligament, cementum, and alveolar bone proper. Small irregularly shaped calcified structures known as cementicles are also found in the periodontal ligament.

Following are the roles of the periodontal ligament:

1. Mechanical functions

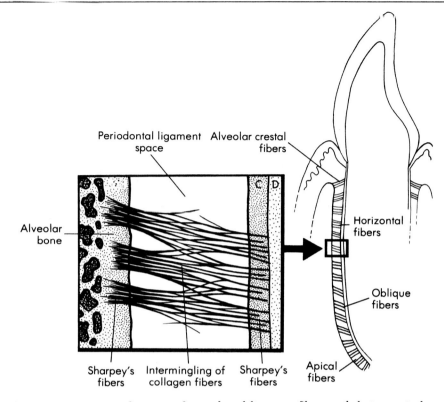

FIGURE 1-10. Principal groups of periodontal ligament fibers and their terminal portions, Sharpey's fibers.

2. Formative function
3. Nutritive function
4. Sensory function

The mechanical functions are to attach the tooth to the bone and provide a cushion that partially absorbs forces directed onto the teeth. In addition, the principal fibers transmit tension forces to the alveolar bone when occlusal forces are generated. The tension is important in maintaining normal bone apposition and trabecular patterns.

The formative function is carried out by the many connective tissue cells that are present. Throughout the life of the tooth cementoblasts are continuously forming cementum, fibroblasts are continually forming collagen, and osteoblasts are forming bone. Without an intact periodontal ligament, continuous deposition of cementum and bone is not possible.

The nutritive function is performed by the blood supply of the periodontal ligament when it carries food products to the cells of the area.

The nerves perform the sensory function. Both pain and proprioceptive receptors are present and play an important role in the monitoring of mandibular function.

The periodontal ligament has also been known as the periodontal membrane. However, since its principal structures and functions resemble those of a ligament more than those of a membrane, the preferred term is *periodontal ligament.*

ALVEOLAR BONE

The alveolar bone is made up of bony processes that project from the basal portions of the mandible and maxilla. These processes are composed principally of cancellous or spongy

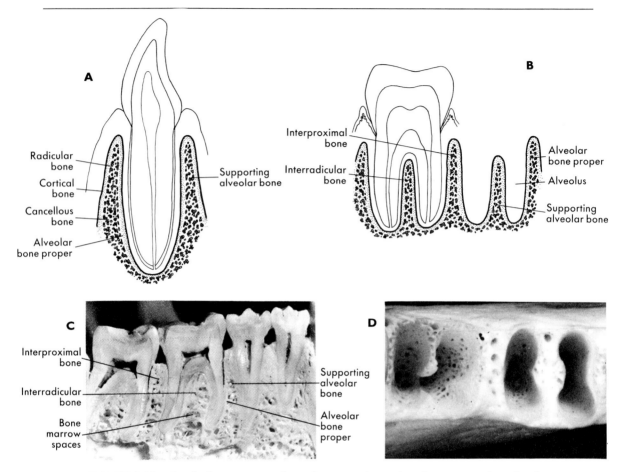

FIGURE I-II. Alveolar bone. **A,** Faciolingual section of a tooth and its surrounding alveolar bone. **B,** Mesiodistal section of a tooth and its surrounding alveolar bone. **C,** Mesiodistal section of posterior teeth and alveolar bone. **D,** Occlusal view of alveoli.

bone covered with a harder outer covering known as cortical bone (Fig. 1-11, A). The alveolar processes form as the teeth develop and erupt into the oral cavity. They do not form unless teeth are present, and following the extraction of teeth they gradually resorb.

The spaces in the alveolar bone that accommodate the roots of the teeth are known as *alveoli* (Fig. 1-11, B). The alveoli are lined with a layer of bone known as the *alveolar bone proper* or the *cribriform plate* (Fig. 1-11, B and C), so called because there are many small holes in which Sharpey's fibers and blood vessels are embedded. This layer of bone shows as a white line on radiographs and is called the *lamina dura*. This layer of bone also covers the crest of the interproximal bone and is known radiographically as the *crestal lamina dura*. The cancellous and cortical bone that surrounds the alveolar bone proper is known as the *supporting alveolar bone* (Fig. 1-11).

The alveolar processes are subdivided into various parts depending on their anatomical relationships to the teeth they surround. The bone located between the roots of adjacent teeth is known as the *interproximal bone* or the

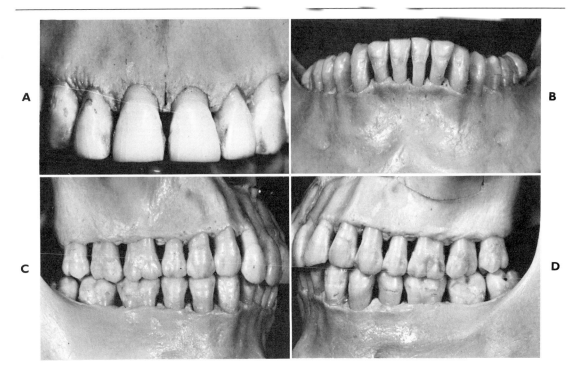

FIGURE 1-12. A, Facial view of maxillary anterior teeth and supporting alveolar bone. Note tapered contours and pyramidal shape of the crestal portion of the interproximal bone. **B,** Facial view of mandibular anterior teeth and supporting bone. **C,** Right posterior teeth and supporting bone. Note more blunted contour of the crestal portion of the interproximal bone. **D,** Left posterior teeth and supporting bone. Note thicker marginal radicular bone in the molar regions.

interdental septum (Fig. 1-11, *B* and *C*). The bone located between the roots of multirooted teeth is known as the *interradicular bone* (Fig. 1-11, *B* and *C*). The alveolar process located on the facial or lingual surfaces of the roots of teeth is known as the *radicular bone* (Figs. 1-11, *A*, 1-12, and 1-13).

In health the alveolar processes surround the roots to within 1 to 2 mm of the cemento-enamel junction. The crest of the interproximal bone is usually more coronally positioned than the adjacent radicular bone (Figs. 1-12 and 1-13). The thickness and contour of the alveolar bone depend primarily on the position of the teeth in the arch and their relationship to one another. Teeth that are labially positioned in the arch will have thin labial radicular bone

and thicker lingual radicular bone (Fig. 1-14). In some instances a portion of the root is not covered with bone. If it is an isolated area, it is known as a *fenestration* (window) (Fig. 1-13, *B*). However, if the bony defect includes the bone margin, it is known as a *dehiscence* (Fig. 1-13, *C*).

In the absence of disease the angle at which the interproximal crestal bone meets the adjacent teeth depends on the positioning of the adjacent teeth. In general the line of the interproximal crestal bone will be parallel to a line drawn between the adjacent cementoenamel junctions. If the teeth have erupted to the same occlusal height, the interproximal bone will be horizontal in contour (Fig. 1-15, *A*). However, if one tooth has tilted or erupted far-

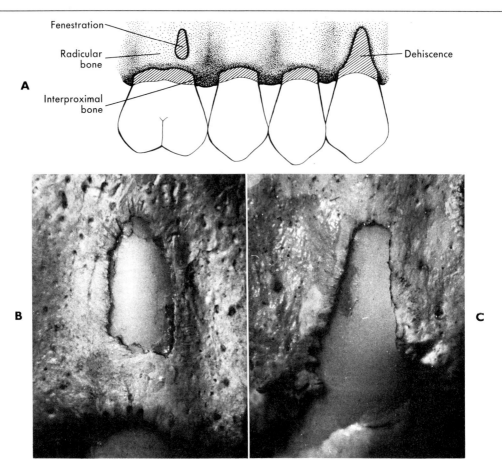

FIGURE 1-13. A, Buccal view of the alveolar process. Note that the crest of the interproximal bone is more coronal than the radicular bone. **B,** Fenestration. **C,** Dehiscence.

ther than the adjacent tooth, the crestal bone will be tilted parallel to the line drawn between the adjacent cementoenamel junctions (Fig. 1-15, *B* and *C*).

The alveolar bone present at any one point in time is the net result of the processes of bone formation and resorption, which take place throughout life. The osteoblast (bone-forming cell) secretes an organic matrix consisting primarily of collagen called *osteoid* (or prebone), which subsequently calcifies to form bone. The osteoblasts that become enmeshed in the bone matrix become *osteocytes*. They are located in *lacunae* (spaces within the bone), which are connected by narrow channels called *canaliculi*. The resorption of bone is thought to be primarily related to the cell known as the *osteoclast*. It is a multinucleated cell found in concavities of bone surfaces called *Howship's lucanae*. In the alveolar bone they are found on the periosteal (outer), endosteal (marrow), or periodontal ligament surfaces of the bone. Even though alveolar bone is a rather sturdy tissue, it is the most labile of all the periodontal tissues, continually being resorbed while new bone is being formed.

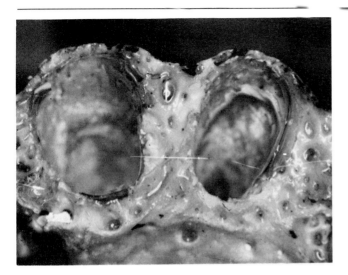

FIGURE 1-14. Two alveoli. Note the relatively thin labial radicular wall of bone and the thicker lingual wall. This is the result of the teeth being positioned more to the labial rather than the lingual aspect of the alveolar process.

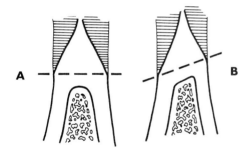

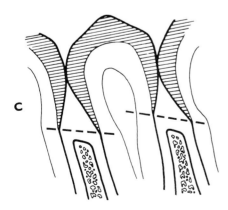

FIGURE 1-15. Mesiodistal sections of the periodontium illustrating that the crestal contour of the interdental bone parallels a line drawn between the cementoenamel junction on adjacent teeth.

CEMENTUM

Cementum is calcified tissue that covers the root of the tooth and provides a means of attachment for the periodontal ligament fibers to the tooth. Cementum is continuously formed on root surfaces that are in contact with the periodontal ligament or gingival fibers. New cementum cannot be formed on root surfaces that have been denuded of their connective tissue attachment because it is formed by cells in the periodontal ligament. Cementum consists of calcified collagen fibers and interfibrillar ground substance. Cementoblasts form the organic matrix known as *cementoid* precementum, which is subsequently calcified to form cementum. Cementum is made up of 45% to 50% inorganic material and 50% to 55% organic matter and water. This composition makes cementum slightly harder than bone. The width of cementum varies from 16 to 60 μm in the coronal half of the root: this is approximately the thickness of a hair. Cementum is much thicker on the apical third of the root, being 150 to 200 μm.

Two types of cementum are seen, *acellular* and *cellular*. The acellular cementum is found principally on the coronal areas of the roots and is characterized by dense layers of calcified collagen fibers separated by growth lines that are areas of calcified interfibrillar material. The layers generally run parallel to the long axis of the tooth.

The cellular cementum is found more commonly in the apical areas of the roots and in the furcation areas of multirooted teeth. Within the mass of cellular cementum are cementocytes located in lacunae. The cementocytes are cementoblasts that have been embedded in the cementum during its formation. They receive their nourishment through canaliculi. Both cellular and acellular cementum function equally well as attachment and covering materials for the root.

The cementoenamel junction is the area of the tooth where the enamel of the anatomical crown ends on the root surface. There can be three different relationships among the enamel, cementum, and dentin in this area. In approximately 60% to 65% of the cases the cementum overlaps the enamel, in about 30% of the cases there is an edge-to-edge meeting of the cementum and the enamel, and in 5% to 10% of the areas the cementum fails to meet the enamel, resulting in exposed dentin. If these areas are exposed by gingival recession or periodontitis, they may be more sensitive than surrounding areas.

SUMMARY

The periodontium consists of four different tissues: gingiva, periodontal ligament, alveolar bone, and cementum. They are anatomically separate, but functionally they all depend on one another in maintaining a viable, healthy supporting structure for the tooth.

SUGGESTED READINGS

Baer PN, and Morris M: Textbook of periodontics, Philadelphia, 1977, JB Lippincott Co, pp 1-63.

Listgarten MA: Electron microscopic study of the junction between surgically denuded root surfaces and regenerated periodontal tissues, J Periodont Res 7:68, 1972.

Schluger S, Yuodelis R, and Page R: Periodontal disease, Philadelphia, 1977, Lea & Febiger, pp 7-55.

Stern, IB: Current concepts of the dentogingival junction: the epithelial and connective tissue attachments to the tooth, J Periodontol 52(9):465, 1981.

Strahan JD, and Waite IM: Color atlas of periodontology, Chicago, 1979, Year Book Medical Publishers, Inc., pp 9-14.

CHAPTER 2
Basic Etiology of Periodontal Disease

Etiology is the science of causes or origins. Etiological factors in relationship to periodontal disease are those factors or agents that in some way cause, modify, or contribute to the development of periodontal tissue injury or destruction. *Periodontal disease* refers to all the diseases of the periodontium; this means that a periodontal disease is any pathological state that involves the supporting tissues of the teeth.

The concept of etiology is important because both the prevention and the treatment of dental diseases depend on a thorough understanding of the relationship between the etiological factors and the pathogenesis of periodontal disease and dental caries.

With the increasing awareness and attention being placed on etiological factors, patient education and plaque control programs are playing a vital role in complete patient care. These programs require the identification of specific etiological factors and the knowledge of how a specific agent can cause the tissue changes characteristic of various periodontal diseases. Prevention, the goal of all health professions, can only be achieved when the causes of specific diseases are identified then eliminated or controlled.

TYPES OF ETIOLOGICAL FACTORS

The primary factor in the etiology of inflammatory periodontal diseases is the accumulation and maturation of bacterial plaque on the teeth near the gingival margin and/or in the sulcus or pocket. However, the patient's periodontal tissue response to the bacteria is influenced by local, immune, and systemic resistance factors. In periodontal health a balance exists between the pathogenicity of the small amounts of bacterial plaque present on the teeth and the patient's resistance. When gingivitis or periodontitis develops, an imbalance exists between the pathological effects of the microorganisms and the ability of the patient's local, immune, and systemic defense mechanisms. Most commonly the imbalance is related to an increase in the number or changes in the types of microorganisms present, but changes in the defense mechanisms also occur that can upset the balance and allow pathological changes to develop with only minimal changes in the plaque.

Local resistance factors include the crevicular fluid, epithelial barriers, and anatomical factors. Immune mechanisms include hypersensitive reactions to the bacteria such as anaphylaxis or immediate hypersensitivity, immune complex reactions, and cytotoxic reactions. Systemic factors are hormonal changes such as pregnancy and blood dyscrasias.

Etiological factors in periodontal disease are usually classified into two broad categories, depending on their specific origin:

I. Local (extrinsic) etiologic factors
   A. Irritating factors
      1. Initiating factor
      2. Predisposing factors
   B. Functional factors
II. Systemic (intrinsic) etiological factors

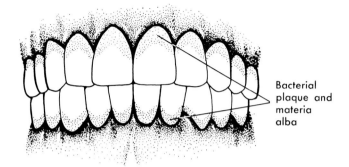

Bacterial
plaque and
materia
alba

FIGURE 2-1. Bacterial plaque and materia alba accumulate most readily on the gingival third of the facial and lingual surfaces of the teeth and on the interproximal surfaces adjacent to the gingiva.

Local factors are those found in the immediate environment of the tissues of the periodontium and can be divided into irritating and functional factors. *Local irritating factors* can further be separated into the *local initiating factor* and *local predisposing factors.* Bacterial plaque is the local initiating factor because it causes gingival inflammation when it accumulates on the teeth adjacent to the gingiva. Predisposing factors such as overhanging margins on restorations create a dentogingival environment that favors the accumulation of bacterial plaque. Local functional factors such as bruxism act by creating occlusal forces that cause destruction of the periodontal ligament and alveolar bone but do not directly affect the inflammatory process. *Systemic factors* are conditions affecting the total body health that also adversely affect the tissues of the periodontium. An example is diabetes mellitus.

ROLE OF ETIOLOGICAL FACTORS

The local, immunological, and systemic factors involved in periodontal disease are definitely interconnected in that together they play a vital role in the etiology of tissue injury or destruction. Today in the field of periodontology controversy still exists over the exact roles of the local and systemic factors and their interassociation in the etiology of periodontal disease.

In most periodontal diseases local factors such as bacterial plaque play the primary role in the etiology of the inflammation and associated tissue destruction; systemic factors such as hormonal changes play the secondary role in that they exaggerate the tissue response to local etiological factors. The systemic factors by themselves do not initiate periodontal changes, but some systemic etiological factors such as ingestion of phenytoin (Dilantin) can play the primary role in causing hyperplastic gingival changes. In this situation local factors play a secondary role by exaggerating the tissue changes initiated by systemic factors. While certain degenerative and hyperplastic gingival tissue changes can be caused by systemic changes, no identified systemic factors are capable of initiating periodontal pocket formation.

LOCAL (EXTRINSIC) ETIOLOGICAL FACTORS

Soft deposits play a role in the etiology of periodontal disease. The effect of these deposits depends on their particular type and their relationship to the gingival tissues (Figs. 2-1 and 2-2). Soft deposits act with several different mechanisms to cause gingival and periodontal inflammation.

  1. Soft deposits are a favorable environment

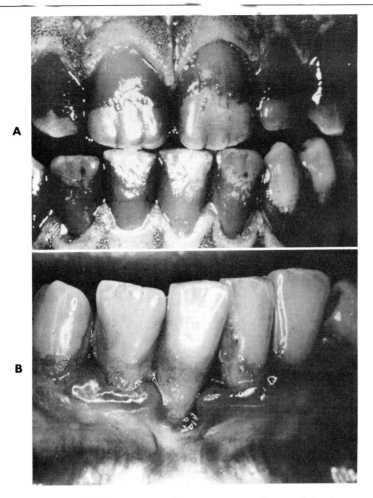

FIGURE 2-2. A, Typical plaque accumulation patterns when oral hygiene measures are withheld for several days. **B,** Long-standing plaque deposits noted at the time of initial examination of this patient with periodontitis.

for the production and growth of microorganisms.

2. Plaque microorganisms invade the gingival tissues and cause inflammation by their production of toxins, enzymes, or antigens (Fig. 2-2).
3. Soft deposits, when mineralized, become calculus (Fig. 2-3).
4. Soft deposits participate in caries production.

Local irritating factors
Initiating factor—bacterial plaque (dental plaque, microbial plaque)

Bacterial plaque (Fig. 2-2) is a complex, tenaciously attached, soft deposit composed of a consistently organized structure of microorganisms, epithelial cells, leukocytes, macrophages, intermicrobial matrix, and water. The intermicrobial matrix of plaque forms from salivary proteins and is believed to hold and unite the

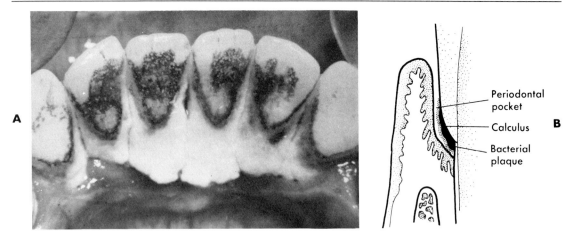

FIGURE 2-3. A, Large supragingival deposits of calculus on the lingual surfaces of mandibular incisors. **B,** Calculus in a periodontal pocket. Note that the plaque on the surface of the calculus is being held in close contact with the gingival sulcular tissues.

plaque bacteria, keeping it firmly adherent to the underlying surface.

Bacterial plaque is usually deposited on a thin bacteria-free film called the *acquired pellicle* (acquired cuticle). This pellicle is colorless and transparent unless stained. The acquired pellicle is a glycoprotein from the saliva, and it will form on a clean tooth surface within minutes. It is firmly adherent to the tooth surface and can be formed on oral appliances and restorations.

Initially and in small amounts bacterial plaque is transparent and therefore not clinically visible. This explains the use of disclosing agents as a means of plaque detection. As plaque goes through a highly complex, sophisticated maturation process by the proliferation and addition of bacteria and bacterial by-products, it becomes visible by its mass and discoloration. Plaque can be removed by mechanical cleaning and accumulates both supragingivally and subgingivally, mostly around the gingival third of the tooth and interproximal areas. Plaque may be deposited on a cleaned tooth surface within 6 hours, with maximal accumulation achieved in approximately 30 days.

Plaque microbiota. The normal oral flora varies from individual to individual. Within the normal flora a counterbalance among the microorganisms exists, with no destructive changes occurring to the periodontal tissues; it is when these organisms lose their natural physiological balance that destructive tissue changes are initiated. Such is the case when microorganisms are allowed to accumulate in large amounts and mature into more pathological forms in bacterial plaque. Bacterial plaque consists of a mixture of diverse microorganisms. The longer plaque remains on the tooth surface, the more types of microorganisms will be present, until the plaque reaches maturity in a few days. The plaque microbiota is extremely complex. Following are genuses of microorganisms representative of the numerous bacteria that are related to the plaque microbiota and its stages of maturation.

1. Gram-positive cocci—*Streptococcus, Staphylococcus*
2. Gram-positive rods—*Lactobacillus, Actinomyces*
3. Gram-negative rods—*Bacteroides, Fusobacterium*

4. Spirochaeta

Microorganisms in the plaque exert their destructive action, causing tissue injury, damage, and disease, by various mechanisms as follows:

1. Production of toxins (exotoxins and endotoxins)
2. Production of enzymes (collagenase and proteases)
3. Production of bacterial antigens
4. Production of bacterial waste products (ammonia, hydrogen sulfide)
5. Invasion of the gingival tissues

All these microbial products act as irritating substances that produce the changes in the periodontal tissues.

The role of bacterial plaque in the etiology of periodontal disease is extremely complex and is not fully established. The results of numerous research projects have indicated that bacterial plaque is the principal etiological agent of inflammatory periodontal diseases. The etiological potential probably depends on the concentration of different types of bacteria and their products in a localized area of the gingival sulcus. This concentration upsets the normal healthy bacteria-host relationship, and disease results.

No definitive statements can be made regarding the rate and location of plaque formation because they vary from individual to individual and from one area of the mouth to another. Microbial activity is related to host resistance. For periodontal health a balance must exist among the oral microorganisms and between the microorganisms and the host. If the resistance of the host is reduced, this balance is disturbed and disease may result. Local host resistance is tissue protection provided by the normal body defense mechanisms, which include the following:

1. Healthy, intact epithelial tissues (the main function of epithelial tissue is protection)
2. Keratinization of the epithelium that covers the oral aspects of the gingiva (gingival sulcular epithelium is not keratinized)
3. Fluids from the gingival sulcus that contain antibodies and provide a "washing-out" effect
4. Antibacterial and self-cleaning action of saliva
5. Use of the muscles of mastication and the tongue, which provide natural cleaning effects

Systemic host resistance involves total body health. Degenerative diseases such as diabetes mellitus can affect the resistance of the tissues. If host resistance is lowered, the periodontal tissues have less defense against the destructive aspects of the chronic inflammatory lesion. Lowered resistance results in accentuated gingival changes and more rapid bone loss.

History and examples of microbial and immunological mechanisms in periodontal diseases. Until 1955 most dentists believed that periodontal disease was caused by calculus. Calculus is yellow or black-green and appears to be irritating the gingiva. It was believed that if the ugly, hard, and rough calculus was removed, the adjacent gingival tissues would heal and oral health would be restored. This belief was one of the fundamentals of dental hygiene methodology for many years. However, between 1955 and 1970 it was shown that calculus was actually mineralized plaque and that the viable bacterial plaque on the surface of calculus rather than the calculus itself was the prime cause of periodontal disease. Although the bacterial plaque was not always visible and was certainly less aesthetically objectionable, it was discovered that regular removal of the bacterial plaque by the patient as well as professional scaling to eliminate the calculus would enhance the restoration and maintenance of gingival health. During this period periodontal diseases were thought to result when the total amount of plaque increased. No individual organisms were identified as causing specific forms of the disease. This idea exemplifies the "nonspecific plaque hypotheses."

In the 1970s another complication was added to the problem. It became apparent that the patient's immunological response to dental plaque plays a major role in the initiation and pathogenesis of periodontal disease. Consistent with this finding, children and young adults were noted to be relatively resistant to periodontal disease while adults became more afflicted with increased age. This increase in periodontal disease with age parallels the decline in the body's ability to respond with strong immunological defense mechanisms. Therefore it was suggested that the patient's immunological defenses might be important in their ability to resist the development of periodontal disease. It may be for this reason that some middle-aged and older patients with periodontal disease do not respond favorably to the conventional therapeutic procedures of plaque control, scaling, and pocket reduction.

In 1975 a new theory added further complexity to the problem. Some researchers believed that they could identify specific bacteria responsible for specific types of periodontal disease. For example, *Actinobacillus actinomycetemcomitans* was isolated and has been shown to be associated with juvenile periodontitis. One strain of this microorganism produces a toxic substance called *leukocidin*, which can destroy white blood cells. White blood cells play a major role in the body's general and immunological defense system against bacteria. Therefore with a reduction in the white blood cells in the gingival tissues less tissue resistance is offered to the microorganisms and their destructive effects are enhanced. This theory is consistent with the rapid destruction of bone found in juvenile periodontitis. The isolation of a specific species of bacteria and identification of its relationship with a particular form of periodontal disease is interpreted by some researchers as support for a concept of bacterial specificity in periodontal disease. However, this concept is still controversial and is in conflict with the more traditional idea that a nonspecific mass of many types of microorganisms is responsible for a number of periodontal tissue changes.

Another proposal for the relationship between plaque microorganisms and periodontal disease is that the bacteria act as "opportunists." In this hypothesis the organisms may be present and play a beneficial or a detrimental role depending upon the circumstances in which they exist. For example, a microorganism may normally be able to prevent the colonization of certain known pathological bacteria, but if allowed to multiply in large numbers may overwhelm the host's immune system and become pathological itself. This is a common occurrence in oral infections and may be true in periodontal diseases.

Today most periodontal researchers, although they may assert the etiological importance of one or two specific subgingival bacterial pathogens, generally agree that the bacteria-host interactions of the mixed subgingival flora and periodontal tissues determine the health or disease of the periodontium. Effective plaque control was the "state of the art" in the prevention and treatment of periodontal disease in the early 1980s. However, further discoveries of the bacteria-host interaction are expanding the surgical, mechanical, and chemical means of treating periodontal diseases and are ushering in newer methods of preventing and controlling periodontal disease.

In discussing the microbial etiology of periodontal disease the characteristics of the sites of bacterial activity, that is, the gingival sulcus and the periodontal pocket, must be considered as well as the nature of the microorganisms present.

The environment of the gingival sulcus is ideal for the growth of oral bacteria. The anatomy of the sulcus makes it relatively resistant to the washing and cleaning action of saliva and the abrasive mechanical activities of the tongue and cheeks during mastication and swallowing. Thus the gingival sulcus becomes a retentive area that forms a relatively stagnant environment for some oral bacteria.

In addition, the oral bacteria that colonize the gingival sulcus are nourished by the protein-rich serum that is filtered through the sulcular epithelium on its way to the oral cavity. This nutritional source is the *gingival fluid*. The gingival fluid contains proteins, carbohydrates, minerals, and vitamins, which foster the growth of the sulcular microflora. As the bacteria in the sulcus cause an inflammatory response in the gingival tissues, the blood vessels enlarge, and an increased amount of gingival fluid is secreted into the sulcus to feed the bacteria that form the subgingival and supragingival plaque.

The unique hydrogen ion concentration (pH) and the oxidation-reduction potential (Eh) of the gingival sulcus are also characteristics of importance to the growth of subgingival bacteria. The acid pH of the gingival sulcus differs from that of the supragingival salivary environment because many plaque bacteria produce acid. The oxidation-reduction potential in the sulcus is low because the supragingival plaque greatly reduces the amount of oxygen-containing air entering the area. The subgingival flora initially contains both aerobic (oxygen-consuming) and anaerobic (growing only in the absence of oxygen) bacteria. However, the oxygen-consuming bacteria quickly use the available oxygen, and the Eh falls rapidly. The low Eh is favorable for the growth of anaerobic oral bacteria. Thus the predominant microbial flora of the periodontal pocket are anaerobic bacteria.

Two other factors further the growth of the subgingival plaque. Once the periodontal lesion is initiated, the dead and dying cells of the periodontal tissues add a new and richer nutritional source to the viable bacteria in the area. Additionally, the metabolic products produced by one group of bacteria may serve as carbon and energy sources for some of the growing anaerobic bacteria in the area. For example, the lactic acid produced by acidogenic bacteria or local tissue cells can be used by the anaerobic *Veillonella* organism as an energy source

and therefore be more pathogenic.

Last, the host defenses of the gingival sulcus differ from the host defenses in other parts of the oral cavity. In the mouth the supragingival flora is exposed to the relatively strong host defenses of the saliva, whereas the subgingival flora encounter the less effective host defenses of the gingival fluid. The defenses of the gingival fluid are weakened as the serum is diluted and passed through the epithelial barrier of the sulcus. If the subgingival bacteria are able to survive and can use the host defense fluids or cells as nutritional sources, they can tip the balance of host defense toward the disease state. The nature of the subgingival microflora in periodontal disease is quite complex, and the number of bacterial species is large. About 84 different species of bacteria have been isolated and cultivated from subgingival plaque at this time, but authorities estimate that about 264 subgingival species may be present in stained smears.

Most of the bacteria in the gingival sulcus are anaerobic. Some of them can be cultivated by the bacterial agar plate or tube method, and these are shown in Table 2-1. At least 12 species are frequently detected in disease sites, and most are anaerobic bacteria.

To help understand the nature of subgingival bacteria, one organism, *Bacteroides gingivalis*, will be discussed in detail. It is one of the most thoroughly studied subgingival plaque anaerobes. It was discovered in 1921 and called *Bacteroides melaninogenicus* because in the presence of blood it produced a black pigment reminiscent of melanin. The organism has been associated with a group of three or four other species in the etiology of periodontal disease in animals. In 1970 the species were subdivided and *Bacteroides gingivalis* was described. It is a nonmotile, nonspore-forming gram-negative anaerobic rod that produces a black pigment when grown on media containing blood, hemin, and vitamin K. It is found in low numbers in the subgingival plaque of individuals with minimal or no periodontal disease, but is

TABLE 2-1

Frequently detected bacterial species from subgingival sites

Species	Incidence (%)	
	Moore et al.*	Newman and Socransky†
Fusobacterium nucleatum	52	86
Fusiform *Bacteroides*	‡	69
Bacteroides gingivalis and other black-pigmented *Bacteroides* (BPB)	26	53
Wolinella recta	‡	53
Actinomyces naeslundii	35	44
Peptostreptococcus micros	‡	33
Eikenella corrodens (vibrio)	‡	30
Streptococcus sanguis	‡	28
Streptococcus intermedius	‡	28
Propionibacterium acnes	‡	23
Actinobacillus actinomycetemcomitans	‡	16
Eubacterium species	12	‡
Capnocytophaga species	<1	‡
Campylobacter species	‡	‡

*Moore WER, Ranney RR, and Holdeman LR: Subgingival flora in periodontal disease. In Genco RJ, and Mergenhagen SE, editors: Host-parasite interactions in periodontal diseases, Washington, 1982, American Society for Microbiology.
†Newman MG, and Socransky SS: J Periodont Res 12:120, 1977.
‡Not available.

recovered in about three quarters of the lesions from patients with advanced periodontal disease. Controversy exists as to whether it accounts for a sizable percentage (20% to 30%) of the total cultivable flora in patients with advanced periodontal disease. It should be emphasized that even though *Bacteroides gingivalis* is very common, it is not recoverable from all advanced periodontal lesions. The organism is capable of causing periodontal disease tissue changes through a variety of products such as an endotoxin, lytic enzymes like collagenase and hyaluronidase, and a number of cytotoxic metabolic products.

Bacteroides gingivalis is representative of the subgingival bacterial flora. While it is a prominent and potentially pathological member of the flora, it is not the specific or only cause of periodontal disease. It is typical of the pathogenic anaerobic subgingival flora and has

therefore been used to explain the microbial aspects in the etiology of periodontal diseases.

While individual microorganisms have not been identified as the definite causes of specific forms of periodontal disease, differences are found in the microbial composition of plaque found in periodontal health and in the various periodontal diseases.

In the periodontally healthy mouth very little dental plaque is found, and it is primarily located supragingivally. The bacterial flora is mainly composed of gram-positive coccal forms, and organisms commonly found are *Streptococcus mitis*, *Streptococcus sanguis*, *Staphylococcus epidermidis*, *Rothia dentocariosa*, *Actinomyces viscosus*, and *Actinomyces naeslundii*. Species of *Neisseria* and *Veillonella* are also sometimes seen. Gram-negative organisms such as *Streptococcus sanguis* and *Fusobacterium naviforme* have been found in healthy sites but comprise only a small proportion of the bacterial flora.

The microflora found in gingivitis vary according to the length of time the plaque and the disease have been present. In the experimental gingivitis model, plaque was allowed to accumulate for 3 weeks without oral hygiene influence. Gingivitis developed, and in addition to the increase in the number of bacteria, the predominant change in the bacterial composition of the supragingival plaque was an increase in the number of *Actinomyces israelii* and *Actinomyces viscosus* and a proportional decrease in the number of gram-positive cocci. This change suggests that the gingivitis developed as a result of changes in the types of organisms as well as an increase in the number of organisms. Changes in the subgingival plaque during chronic gingivitis include a shift to more gram-negative microflora. *Eikenella corrodens, Fusobacterium nucleatum,* and *Capnocytophaga gingivalis* have been shown to be elevated in this type of gingivitis.

With acute necrotizing ulcerative gingivitis the microflora is composed primarily of fusiform bacilli and spirochetes. These organisms are capable of invading the epithelium and the connective tissue of the gingiva. Studies have also shown the following microorganisms in this condition: *Bacteroides intermedius, Treponema, Selenomonas,* and *Fusobacterium nucleatum.* Gingivitis during pregnancy has been shown to have an increase in the proportions of *Bacteroides melaninogenicus* subsp. *intermedius* and *Capnocytophaga.* The increase in these organisms is considered to be related to increased plasma levels of estrogen and progesterone.

In periodontitis the subgingival plaque becomes more complex, and there is a predominance of gram-negative anaerobic organisms. The microflora vary according to the type of periodontitis. In prepubertal periodontitis, which severely affects the primary dentition, the microflora is characterized by the presence of *Actinobacillus actinomycetemcomitans* pri-

marily along with *Selenomonas sputigena, Bacteroides intermedius,* and *Eikenella corrodens.*

In juvenile periodontitis, which is characterized by rapid destruction of the periodontal tissues around more than one tooth in the permanent dentition, there are relatively small amounts of supragingival plaque and calculus and the most commonly found organism is *Actinobacillus actinomycetemcomitans.* Other organisms found in this condition include *Capnocytophaga sputigena, Eikenella corrodens, Fusobacterium nucleatum, Bacteroides capillus,* and *Eubacterium brachy.*

Rapidly progressing periodontitis is an aggressive form of periodontal disease that usually affects young adults 20 to 35 years old. The microflora of this condition is not as specific as juvenile periodontitis but has been described as having elevated proportions of *Bacteroides gingivalis, Bacteroides intermedius, Bacteroides forsythus, Actinobacillus actinomycetemcomitans Eikenella corrodens,* and *Wolinella recta.*

Adult periodontitis is the most common form of periodontitis. It is characterized by amounts of plaque and calculus that correlate with the severity of the disease and usually begins after the age of 35 years. The subgingival plaque in this disease tends to be very complex, and the following types of organisms have elevated proportions: gram-negative, anaerobic, capnophilic, and motile. No one organism has been identified as the principal pathogen in adult periodontitis; most likely it is caused by several organisms. Organisms typically associated with this condition are *Bacteroides gingivalis, Bacteroides intermedius, Bacteroides forsythus, Bacteroides capillus, Eikenella corrodens, Fusobacterium nucleatum, Wolinella recta, Selenomonas sputigena, Eubacterium timidum, Eubacterium brachy, Peptostreptococcus micros,* and *spirochetes.*

In recent years efforts have been made to determine periodontal disease activity (progressing resorption of bone and apical movement of the periodontal attachment levels) through the identification of certain microorganisms in the gingival sulcus or pocket. Several investigators feel that there is a correlation between the presence of *Actinobacillus actinomycetemcomitans*, *Bacteroides gingivalis*, and *Bacteroides intermedius* and active disease. Laboratory tests are available to identify the levels of these organisms in a practical manner.

In "refractory" adult periodontitis the disease does not respond to therapy, and the subgingival plaque has elevated proportions of *Actinobacillus actinomycetemcomitans*, *Bacteroides gingivalis*, and *Bacteroides intermedius*.

In contrast to earlier observations, microorganisms are now found to be invading the epithelial and connective tissue areas of the gingiva in acute necrotizing ulcerative gingivitis and juvenile and adult periodontitis.

In addition to producing substances that directly affect the periodontal tissues, the microorganisms in dental plaque also have the ability to produce immunomodulating agents. These agents have the capabilities of either enhancing or suppressing the immune responses of the body. For example, the leukocidin produced by *Actinobacillus actinomycetemcomitans* destroys immunologically important white blood cells in patients with juvenile periodontitis and thereby plays an important role in the etiology and pathogenesis of the disease. The cells that are destroyed are polymorphonuclear neutrophils (PMNs) and macrophages. The polymorphonuclear neutrophils provide an important local host defense against microorganisms and their noxious products, while the macrophages play an important role in the patient's general immune defense response.

In adult periodontitis the interaction between bacterial substances and various immunological host defense mechanisms resulting in destruction of the soft and hard tissues of the periodontium has been studied extensively during the past 10 years and found to be extremely complex. One of the strongest implications of the role of the immune response in the pathogenesis of periodontal disease is the predominance of lymphocytes and plasma cells in the gingival tissues of patients with adult human periodontitis. Lymphocytes and plasma cells are two of the three major cell types involved in the immune response. The third cell type, the mononuclear cell or macrophage, while not predominant in periodontal diseased tissues, has also been associated with periodontal disease processes, particularly when stimulated by bacterial antigens. Thus it is strongly suggested that the immune systems of the body are intimately involved with the cellular and tissue changes seen in periodontal disease.

In addition to the cellular characteristics just mentioned, the following key observations have been made in studying the effects of oral bacteria on immune cells. First, preparations of bacteria from periodontal pockets have been shown to activate antibody-forming B lymphocytes to produce immunoglobulins (antibodies) that are not specifically related to a specific activating bacteria. Second, the majority of the immunoglobulins present in periodontally diseased tissues do not exhibit specificity for bacterial antigenic determinants of periodontal pocket bacteria. Third, immune complexes are not found in affected periodontal tissues. These three characteristics are typical of an antibody response to many bacteria, not just a specific organism.

Despite this rather nonspecific response in the gingival tissues, the activation of peripheral (circulating) blood lymphocytes from patients with adult periodontitis becomes enhanced during successful periodontal treatment. The serum of these patients contains high measures of antibody that is specific for antigens of periodontal pocket bacteria. This suggests that in these patients B lymphocytes have been activated that produce antibodies specific for subgingival bacterial antigens. Research in experimental animals suggests that this antibody may be protective and help prevent periodontal tissue destruction. An example of this protection is seen in patients with juvenile periodontitis who exhibit high levels of antibody to the anti genic determinants of *Actinobacillus actino-mycetemcomitans*, which is commonly found in this disease.

Controversy exists concerning the activation of macrophages by antigenic components of subgingival bacteria. One group of investigators claims that bacteria from patients with periodontal disease activate macrophages to a greater extent than those from healthy patients. The activated macrophages produce substances called *monokines* that modulate the immune and inflammatory responses. One of these responses is the proliferation of lymphocytes. However, another group of investigators claims no correlation between the activation of macrophages by dental plaque bacteria and lymphocyte proliferation.

Polymorphonuclear neutrophils are usually the defense cells found in acute inflammation and are gradually replaced by macrophages. The roles of these phagocytic cells in chronic periodontal diseases are of great interest because they are capable of producing substances that can destroy periodontal tissues.

Of particular interest in periodontitis is the fact that certain white blood cells can be activated by products of dental plaque to produce a substance known as the *osteoclast-activating factor*. The osteoclast is the principal cell involved in bone resorption.

A detailed description of the immunology of periodontal disease is beyond the scope of this textbook. For more details consult the Suggested Readings at the end of the chapter.

Predisposing factors

Materia alba. Materia alba is a visible, soft deposit consisting of microorganisms, leukocytes, salivary proteins, desquamated epithelial cells, and food particles. Like bacterial plaque, materia alba accumulates on teeth, restorations, dental appliances, and the gingiva. Unlike plaque, materia alba is less adherent and can be removed by the application of a forceful water spray. Materia alba does not have the or-

ganized microbial structure of bacterial plaque, and yet evidence indicates that materia alba acts as a favorable environment for the production and growth of diverse microorganisms with pathological potential to cause gingival inflammation.

Food debris (retention and impaction). *Food debris* consists of particles of food retained in the oral cavity and should be differentiated from food impaction. In itself food debris does not appear to cause gingival irritation even though it contains bacteria. Food debris is easier to remove than plaque and materia alba; removal is often accomplished by physiological action.

Orthodontic appliances provide an excellent vehicle for food and plaque retention by creating a dentogingival environment that requires special techniques for effective plaque control.

Food impaction is the forceful wedging of food between the gingiva and the tooth (Fig. 2-4). It occurs primarily in interproximal areas, but can also occur on the facial and lingual surfaces of teeth in poor occlusal relationships (deep overbite). Interproximal food impaction can be caused by the improper location and relationship of proximal contact points, irregularities in tooth position, or reduced height and blunted contour of the interdental gingiva.

Food impaction and retention may have in-

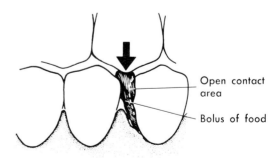

FIGURE 2-4. Forceful wedging of food between two teeth can irritate the gingiva and create an ideal environment for the accumulation of dental plaque.

jurious effects on periodontal tissues: (1) food particles create a favorable environment for plaque accumulation, and (2) food impaction acts as a direct mechanical irritant to the tissues.

Food consistency. The type of diet can influence the rate of plaque formation. A diet of soft, sticky foods produces more bacterial plaque because the soft food clings to the tooth and thereby acts as a favorable environment for plaque accumulation and retention. Frequent exposures to retentive sugars or sweets are particularly harmful. Refined sugars such as sucrose provide substrates for bacterial growth and synthesis of extracellular polysaccharides (glucans) that enhance plaque formation and adherence to teeth. On the other hand, foods of firm, fibrous character enhance oral clearance of food particles or debris.

Dental stains. Dental stains are pigmented deposits on the tooth surface. They are often the results of pigmentation of the acquired pellicle by chromogenic bacteria, food, or chemical agents. Stain associated with the use of chlorhexidine as a mouthwash is an example of the latter. Dental stains may lead to tissue irritation by creating a rough tooth surface, which contributes to plaque accumulation and retention.

Calcified deposits—calculus (Fig. 2-3). Calculus is bacterial plaque that has been mineralized. It can be formed on all tooth surfaces and dental prostheses. Because calculus is calcified mineralized plaque, it begins with the development of plaque. Therefore if plaque must be present for calculus to form, controlling calculus deposition begins with plaque control. Calculus is classified according to its location and source of the calcium into two types, supragingival (salivary) and subgingival (serumnal).

Supragingival calculus is usually light in color and chalky in consistency. The mineral source for supragingival deposits is primarily the saliva. Therefore the deposits are sometimes referred to as salivary calculus. These deposits are more prominent on the lingual sur-

faces of the mandibular anterior teeth and the buccal surfaces of the maxillary molars, which are adjacent to the major salivary ducts.

Subgingival calculus is usually darker in color and more dense. The main source of mineralization for this type of deposit is considered to be the blood, so it is referred to as serumnal calculus.

The exact role calculus plays in the etiology of periodontal disease is difficult to determine, although it is significant. Calculus is usually if not always covered by a layer of nonmineralized plaque. The primary destructive action of calculus is that it acts as a holding mechanism for the nonmineralized surface plaque. The underlying calculus acts as a nidus for the accumulation of the surface plaque and keeps the plaque in direct contact with the tissues.

Caries. Caries is the pathological destruction of the tooth structure. This loss of tooth structure does not in itself cause periodontal disease, but it acts as a favorable environment for the accumulation and retention of soft deposits (Fig. 2-5).

Smoking and tobacco. The stain, heat, and smoke created by cigars, pipes, and cigarettes may lead to deleterious gingival changes. Chewing tobacco can also produce destruction of the gingival tissues. Research evidence indicates an increased prevalence and severity of periodontal disease in people who smoke or chew tobacco. Smokers may also exhibit an increase in plaque accumulation.

Improper oral hygiene. Poor oral hygiene is responsible to a large degree for the accumulation of local deposits that cause tissue destruction. Proper oral hygiene has a twofold effect on the tissues of the oral cavity.

1. The primary role of oral hygiene is the removal of soft deposits on the tooth structure, thereby preventing local irritation and bacterial proliferation.
2. Gingival stimulation may play a role in increasing gingival tone, surface keratinization, and gingival vascularity.

Oral hygiene techniques can have destruc-

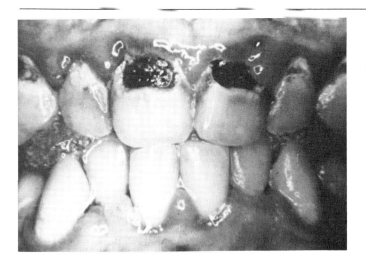

FIGURE 2 5. Note the carious lesions on the facial surfaces of the maxillary incisors, which create rough surfaces that favor plaque accumulation.

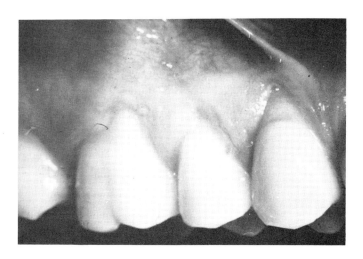

FIGURE 2-6. Cervical abrasion and gingival recession related to toothbrush trauma in a 16-year-old boy.

tive effects if used improperly. Toothbrush trauma caused by vigorous brushing in a horizontal direction or in any incorrect harmful fashion may lead to destruction of gingival tissues because it acts as an agent of irritation (Fig. 2-6). Improper use of dental floss and interdental stimulators may also result in destruction of the tissues of the interdental gingiva, laceration of tissues, and alteration of the ideal gingival contour.

Deficient dental treatment. Following are predisposing etiological factors created by inadequate dental restorations and prostheses:

1. Overhanging margins of dental restorations (Fig. 2-7)
2. Open interproximal contacts of dental restorations
3. Deficient margins on crowns, jackets, and synthetic porcelain restorations
4. Fixed and removable prostheses adapted improperly
5. Overcontoured dental restorations and pontics creating excessive buccolingual contours and inadequate interproximal embrasure spaces (Fig. 2-8)
6. Clasps of partial dentures that retain

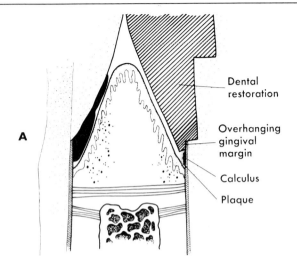

A

- Dental restoration
- Overhanging gingival margin
- Calculus
- Plaque

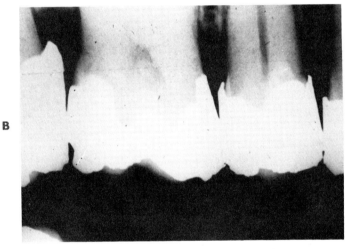

B

FIGURE 2-7. **A,** Overhanging gingival margin of a restoration that creates an ideal environment for plaque accumulation. It is difficult to remove the plaque with normal oral hygiene devices from the area just apical to the excess restorative material. **B,** Radiographic illustration of overhanging gingival margins of the restorations.

plaque, impinge on the gingiva, or exert excessive occlusal forces

These conditions are considered predisposing factors because they do the following:

1. Interfere with proper oral hygiene techniques
2. Lead to food impaction and retention
3. Create areas favoring plaque accumulation
4. Displace the gingival tissue
5. Create excessive occlusal forces

Local functional factors
Unreplaced missing teeth

The sequelae of missing teeth may have injurious effects on the periodontium. Missing teeth can lead to mesial drifting, tilting, and extrusion of teeth. These alterations in the position and functional relationships of teeth can result in increased plaque formation, food impaction, soft deposit retention, and occlusal disharmonies.

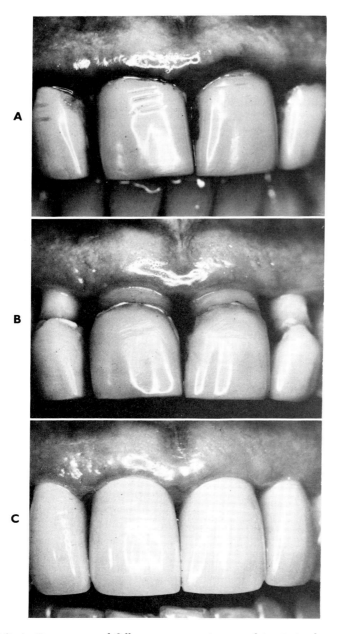

FIGURE 2-8. A, Overcontoured full crown restorations resulting in inadequate interdental embrasure space, excessive retention of plaque, gingival inflammation, and pocket formation in 31-year-old woman. **B,** Same patient following partial recontouring of crowns and periodontal surgery to create access for more adequate plaque control. **C,** Same patient following the placement of new crowns with contours and gingival margins that provide access for adequate plaque control.

Malocclusion

A malocclusion may act as an etiological factor by causing tilting occlusal forces and by precipitating parafunctional occlusal habits. Other anatomical irregularities such as high muscle and frenum attachments can create an environment more conducive to plaque retention, interfere with normal home care procedures, and reduce or eliminate the attached gingiva.

Dental occlusion

The tissues of the periodontium depend on occlusal forces generated by the functioning occlusion for the stimulation they need to remain healthy. When these forces exceed physiological limits, the tissues undergo injury. This injury is referred to as *occlusal trauma*. Insufficient forces caused by missing teeth or malocclusion also cause pathological atrophic changes known as *disuse periodontal atrophy*.

Evidence indicates that excessive occlusal forces cause destruction by crushing and tearing the tissues in a confined area—the periodontal ligament space. Therefore they do not directly affect the gingival tissues.

Excessive occlusal forces cannot cause inflammation, gingivitis, or periodontitis. However, by causing degenerative changes in the deep periodontal structures, the inflammatory process in the overlying gingival tissues is allowed to spread apically more rapidly and result in more severe periodontal tissue destruction.

Parafunctional occlusal habits

Certain habits, such as bruxism (grinding teeth), clenching and clamping the teeth, and chewing on objects such as pipes and pencils, create excessive forces on the tissues of the periodontium. These habits are referred to as parafunctional because they are not part of the normal function of the occlusion. If the degree and duration of these habits are strong enough to create forces that exceed the adaptive capacity of the periodontium, occlusal trauma can develop.

Tongue thrusting

Another habit that has injurious effects is forceful thrusting of the tongue against either the posterior or the anterior teeth. This condition is called *tongue thrusting*, and it can act as a predisposing factor in periodontal disease. It causes interference with the normal self-cleaning action of the tongue. It places teeth in abnormal positions in the dental arch.

Mouth breathing

Mouth breathing caused by incomplete lip closure or nasal obstruction may exaggerate a plaque-caused inflammatory reaction in the gingival tissues (Fig. 2-9). The exact mechanism of injury to the cells is unknown. Evidence indicates that the injury results from the dehydrating effect of constant wetting and drying of the gingiva.

• • •

Following is an outline of local etiological factors in periodontal disease:

I. Local irritating factors
   A. Initiating factor—bacterial (dental) plaque
   B. Predisposing factors
     1. Materia alba
     2. Food debris and retention
     3. Dental stains
     4. Calculus
     5. Caries
     6. Smoking and tobacco
     7. Food impactions
     8. Deficient dental treatment
     9. Improper oral hygiene
     10. Soft, sticky foods (food consistency)
II. Local functional factors
   A. Missing teeth
   B. Malocclusion
   C. Tongue thrusting, mouth breathing
   D. Parafunctional habits
   E. Traumatogenic occlusion

Obviously any number of local factors may be present and active simultaneously. This fact contributes to the complexity of the etiology.

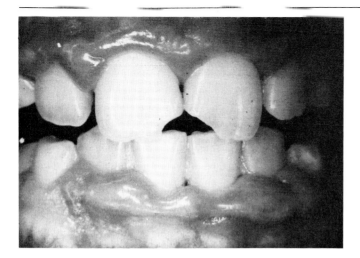

FIGURE 2-9. Exaggerated gingival enlargement in an 11-year-old boy related to a habit of mouth breathing and the hormonal change of puberty.

SYSTEMIC (INTRINSIC) ETIOLOGICAL FACTORS

Systemic factors, conditions affecting the entire body's health, can have adverse effects on the tissues of the periodontium.

Periodontal tissue manifestations of systemic conditions vary according to the specific disease, individual response, and existing local factors.

Systemic factors involved in the etiology of periodontal disease are definitely interrelated with local factors. It is generally accepted that systemic factors by themselves cannot cause an inflammatory response of the gingiva. However, these factors can play a role in the etiology by lowering the resistance of the periodontal tissues, making them more susceptible to the effects of the local factors.

The systemic factors that play a role in periodontal disease can be classified under the following categories:

1. Endocrine (hormonal) factors
2. Nutritional disorders and deficiencies
3. Drugs
4. Psychological (emotional) factors
5. Heredity
6. Metabolic diseases
7. Hematological disturbances and diseases

Endocrine (hormonal) factors

Puberty, pregnancy, and menopause are three situations in which the body undergoes hormonal changes that create endocrine imbalances. Clinical as well as histological research indicates that these hormonal changes can have a marked effect on the gingival tissue changes initiated by local factors. The exact mechanism of the gingival involvement is unknown. The classic symptoms associated with these conditions are described in Chapter 4.

Nutritional disorders and deficiencies

All cells of the body depend on essential nutrients for their proper function and integrity. A variety of negative effects can occur if the body tissues are deprived of these nutrients. Nutritional deficiencies can result from the absence of one or more essential components from the diet. The precise effects of nutritional deficiencies on the periodontal tissues are still under research and experimentation.

Although inflammatory periodontal disease is not the result of a primary nutritional deficiency, nutrient imbalances can amplify the harmful effects of local irritants and modify the progression of the disease. The connective and epithelial tissues of the periodontium depend on at least 50 essential nutrients for normal growth, function, and maintenance. Deficiencies or toxicities of one or more of the nutrients can alter tissue integrity and compromise resistive powers in combating the effects of local irritants.

Clinical symptoms of severe deficiencies in protein, calories, B-complex vitamins, iron, zinc, and vitamins A and C include specific lesions and alterations in color and topography of the oral mucosa and tongue. In animal studies, calcium deficiency, especially with high phosphorus intakes, and deficiencies in vitamin D and magnesium have been shown to adversely affect the formation and integrity of mineralized tissues of the periodontium. Also, nutrients are essential for maintaining cellular defense mechanisms of antibodies and white blood cells. Both epidemiological and experimental studies have demonstrated that severe deficiencies in vitamins A, C, pyridoxine, and pantothenic acid as well as protein and iron result in decreased antibody response and lowered phagocytic activity.

While no substantiated evidence exists that nutritional factors initiate periodontal disease or pocket formation, nutritional imbalances, even at a marginal level, will influence the response of the periodontium to local irritants, infection, and tissue repair. This is particularly true of tissues with a high cellular turnover rate, such as those found in the gingival sulcus and the alveolar process.

Drugs

Phenytoin is an anticonvulsant drug used in the treatment and control of epilepsy. In about 50% of the patients receiving this medication the gingival tissues become markedly enlarged. Cyclosporine, nifedipine, and diltiazem are other drugs associated with gingival hyperplasia.

The use of contraceptive medication has been shown to increase the rate of flow of the gingival fluid and to accentuate the gingival inflammatory reaction to local irritants.

Psychological (emotional) factors

The psychological stability of an individual is an important but difficult etiological factor to identify. All individuals at one time or another have experienced the physical effects of anxiety, stress, tension, fatigue, and worry.

These conditions may affect the periodontium by altering the tissue metabolism and lowering the host resistance to local irritation—as with acute necrotizing ulcerative gingivitis—or they may stimulate such habits as grinding or clenching of teeth, thereby causing occlusal trauma.

Heredity

The role that heredity plays in the development of inflammatory periodontal disease is not clear. Certain advanced cases of periodontitis, such as juvenile periodontitis, have familial tendencies; however, because of the extremely high incidence of gingivitis and periodontitis in the adult population and in view of the complexity of the etiological factors in periodontal disease, it is difficult to single out the exact role of any one factor.

One condition resulting in a severe overgrowth of the gingival tissues is thought to be related to hereditary factors and is termed familial or hereditary gingival enlargement.

Metabolic diseases

Diabetes mellitus is a chronic disease involving an insulin deficiency. The disease is characterized by an excess of sugar in the blood and urine caused by an insufficiency in carbohydrate metabolism.

In uncontrolled states diabetes is characterized by protein breakdown and lowered resistance to infection, producing a higher susceptibility to infection, slower healing rate, vascular deficiencies, and an increase in the severity of inflammatory reactions.

Because of their lowered resistance, oral tissues are more susceptible to the local irritants found in the oral cavity. Research indicates that diabetes may accentuate the resorption of bone in periodontitis. However, it has never been shown to initiate pocket formation.

Hematological disturbances and diseases

The vascular system is the vehicle by which the body receives all the nutrients and substances needed to keep the cells functioning properly. Any hematological disorder can impair this function and cause tissue injury. Like every other body tissue, the periodontium also depends on proper blood flow and composition.

Leukemia is a disease of unknown origin characterized by rapid, abnormal proliferation of white blood cells in the blood-forming organs. Tissue disturbances associated with leukemia occur most frequently in the acute monocytic type. Leukemic changes are many and varied. Most of the changes associated with leukemia result from the severely lowered resistance of the tissues to infection. The gingival inflammatory reaction to local irritants in a patient with leukemia is extremely exaggerated.

Anemia is a condition in which red blood cells are reduced in number or deficient in structure. Several types and causes of anemia are known. The oral manifestations of anemia depend on the type and severity of the conditions. The gingiva may appear quite pale. The relationship of anemia to periodontal disease is not specific, however.

• • •

Following is a summary of systemic (intrinsic) factors:

 I. Endocrine (hormonal) factors
   A. Puberty
   B. Pregnancy
   C. Menopause
 II. Nutritional disorders and deficiencies
   A. Vitamin deficiencies
   B. Protein deficiencies
   C. Malnutrition
 III. Drugs
   A. Phenytoin
   B. Contraceptive medication
 IV. Psychological (emotional) factors
   A. Stress
   B. Tension
   C. Fatigue
   D. Anxiety
 V. Heredity
 VI. Metabolic disease—diabetes mellitus
 VII. Hematological disturbances and diseases
   A. Leukemia
   B. Anemia
   C. Hemophilia
   D. Infectious mononucleosis

Obviously any number of systemic factors may be present and active simultaneously. This fact contributes to the complexity of the etiology.

The exact effects of systemic conditions on the periodontium will be discussed in the chapters on specific periodontal diseases.

SUGGESTED READINGS

Baer PN, and Morris ML: Textbook of periodontics, Philadelphia, 1977, JB Lippincott Co, pp 64-95.

Bastiaan RJ, and Waite IM: Effects of tobacco smoking on plaque development and gingivitis, J Periodontol 49:480, 1978.

Carranza F: Glickman's clinical periodontology, ed 5, Philadelphia, 1979, WB Saunders Co, pp 354-541.

Hurt WC: Periodontics in general practice, Springfield, Ill, 1976, Charles C Thomas, Publisher, pp 85-100.

Moore WER, Ranney RR, and Holdeman LR: Subgingival flora in periodontal disease. In Genco RJ, and Nergenhagen SE, editors: Host-parasite interactions in periodontal diseases, Washington, 1982, American Society for Microbiology.

Newman MG, and Sanz M: Oral microbiology with emphasis on etiology. In Perspectives on oral antimicrobial therapeutics, Littleton, Mass, 1987, PSG Publishing, Inc.

Newman MF, and Socransky SS: Predominant cultivable microbiota in periodontosis, J Periodont Res 12:120, 1977.

Roitt I, and Lehner T: Immunology of oral diseases, London, 1980, Blackwell Scientific Publications, Ltd, Chapter 13.

CHAPTER 3
Classification of Periodontal Diseases

There is no widely accepted classification of periodontal diseases because of the variations and complexities of the etiology and pathogenesis of conditions affecting the periodontal tissues. However, as an aid to understanding the different forms of periodontal diseases the following classification is provided. It is based primarily on the tissues affected, but the conditions listed also vary according to their etiological factors and types of pathological tissue changes.

I. Conditions affecting the gingiva only
   A. Acute gingivitis
   B. Chronic gingivitis
   C. Gingival abscess
   D. Allergic gingivitis
   E. Eruption gingivitis
   F. Pericoronitis
   G. Acute primary herpetic gingivostomatitis
   H. Gingivitis associated with pregnancy
   I. Gingivitis associated with puberty
   J. Gingivitis associated with vitamin C deficiency
   K. Gingivitis associated with leukemia
   L. Desquamative gingivitis
   M. Gingival enlargement related to
      1. Inflammation
      2. Hormonal changes
      3. Blood dyscrasias
      4. Medications
      5. Familial characteristics
      6. Mouth breathing
      7. Neoplasias
II. Conditions affecting the periodontal ligament, cementum, and alveolar bone in addition to the gingiva or alone

A. Periodontitis
   1. Prepubertal
   2. Juvenile
   3. Rapidly progressing
   4. Adult
   5. Associated with acquired immune deficiency syndrome (AIDS)
B. Occlusal trauma
C. Periodontal recession
D. Disuse periodontal atrophy

For the purpose of indicating the type and severity of periodontal disease for a patient on a dental insurance reporting form, the following classification is recommended by the American Dental Association:

Type I   Gingivitis—shallow pockets, no bone loss
Type II   Early periodontitis—moderate pockets, minor to moderate bone loss, satisfactory topography
Type III Moderate periodontitis—moderate to deep pockets, moderate to severe bone loss, unsatisfactory topography
Type IV   Advanced periodontitis—deep pockets, severe bone loss, advanced mobility patterns (usually cases involving missing teeth and reconstruction)

CHAPTER 4
Gingivitis

Gingivitis is categorized as follows:

I. Chronic gingivitis
II. Chronic gingivitis modified by systemic factors
    A. Vitamin C deficiency
    B. Leukemia
    C. Puberty
    D. Pregnancy
III. Gingivitis associated with mouth breathing
IV. Allergic gingivitis
V. Desquamative gingivitis
VI. Acute gingival conditions
    A. Acute necrotizing ulcerative gingivitis
    B. Acute primary herpetic gingivostomatitis
    C. Gingivitis in children

INFLAMMATION

Gingivitis is an inflammatory condition of the gingiva and the most common type of gingival disease. Inflammation is the normal response of living tissues to injury and is the primary response of periodontal tissues to irritation; therefore the majority of periodontal diseases are inflammatory in nature. Inflammation is a defense mechanism against injury. In periodontal disease the injury results primarily from the invasion of microorganisms and their microbial products into the gingival tissues. The body seeks to neutralize or destroy the microbial irritants as well as to prepare for tissue repair and healing. However, during the neutralization process tissue destruction occurs as a result of certain associated immunological, chemical, and cellular changes. Immunological mechanisms are commonly considered to be defense responses by the body to the invasion of foreign substances (sensitizing antigens) such as bacteria or viruses. However, immune reactions are also capable of causing tissue destruction by precipitating certain types of overreactions or so-called hypersensitivities. Immunopathological changes (tissue damage) can occur when the tissues of a sensitized person are subsequently exposed to the sensitizing antigens. At least four types of hypersensitivity reactions are important in periodontal disease: anaphylactic, cytotoxic, immune complex, and delayed or cell-mediated hypersensitivity reactions.

In addition to sensitizing antigens, antibodies are also an important component of many immunological reactions. Antibodies are serum proteins classified as immunoglobulins. They are produced by plasma cells, which in turn are lymphocytes that have been transformed as a result of being challenged by antigens.

The anaphylactic type of hypersensitivity involves an antigen reacting with an antibody fixed to a mast cell. The result is the release of substances from the mast cell that have the capability of inducing periodontal tissue damage. Histamine, one of the substances released, is considered to be an important factor in causing vascular changes in inflammation.

The cytotoxic reactions involve antibodies reacting directly with antigens tightly bound to cells. Cell lysis (destruction) and increased synthesis of lysosomal enzymes by polymorphonuclear leukocytes are two examples of changes related to this type of hypersensitivity. Lysosomal enzymes are capable of causing tissue damage.

The immune complex (Arthus) type reactions occur when high levels of antigens are present and antigen-antibody complexes precipitate within and surround small blood vessels, causing isolated areas of tissue damage in the immediate environment of the reaction. Tissue changes may include inflammation, hemorrhage, and tissue necrosis, which are all considered to be related to the release of lysosomal enzymes from polymorphonuclear leukocytes.

Cell-mediated immunity or delayed hypersensitivity is based on the interaction of antigens with the surfaces of lymphocytes. It has been shown under laboratory conditions that lymphocytes sensitized by dental plaque antigens undergo size and functional changes that result in a chronic accumulation of lymphocytes and macrophages, along with the formation of biologically active substances known as *lymphokines*. The latter can affect the activities of macrophages, fibroblasts, and osteoclasts, which are all important in the pathogenesis of periodontal disease.

To establish the correct diagnosis, treatment and prevention of a specific gingivitis, it is necessary to differentiate between inflammatory and other pathological processes that may be present.

Inflammation can play two roles in periodontal disease:

1. Primary role—the inflammatory mechanism is the first and only pathological change present in the tissues. This is the most common way inflammation is manifested in gingival disease (for example, chronic gingivitis).
2. Secondary role—the inflammatory changes play a secondary role in producing the clinical symptoms of a disease that is produced primarily by a systemically caused noninflammatory process. For example, inflammation commonly complicates desquamative gingivitis, which evidence indicates is a degenerative condition brought about by systemic causes. In this situation the primary pathological tissue changes are considered to be degenerative and the inflammation simply exaggerates the clinical symptoms of the disease.

Following are terms used to describe the clinical characteristics of gingivitis:

I. Type of inflammatory reaction
   A. Acute—characterized by rapid onset, severe symptoms, and short duration
   B. Chronic—characterized by persistence, with extremely slow progression over a long period; most common type of gingivitis
II. Extent of inflammatory reaction
   A. Localized—involving the gingiva of a single tooth or group of teeth
   B. Generalized—involving the gingiva of the entire mouth
III. Distribution of inflammatory reaction
   A. Papillary—affecting the interdental gingiva and often extending into the adjacent portion of the marginal gingiva; changes of the interdental gingiva are usually early indicators of gingivitis
   B. Marginal—affecting the gingival margin and possibly also involving part of the attached gingiva contiguous with the marginal gingiva
   C. Diffuse—affecting the papillary, marginal, and attached gingiva

CHRONIC CONDITIONS
Chronic gingivitis
Definition

Chronic gingivitis is a disease in which the gingiva is affected by a chronic inflammatory process. It is the most common type of gingivitis (Fig. 4-1).

Clinical characteristics

Gingival color. The color changes associated with chronic gingivitis begin in the interdental and marginal gingiva and spread to the attached gingiva. The color change starts as a slight redness, and as the chronic inflammatory process increases, the color changes to bluish red and deep blue.

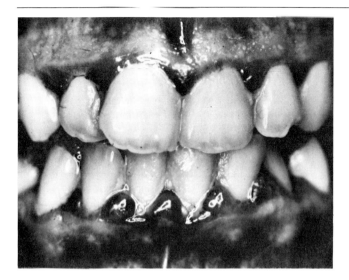

FIGURE 4-1. Chronic gingivitis in a 22-year-old woman. Note the color and contour changes in the marginal and interdental gingiva.

Gingival contour. Chronic gingivitis originates as a slight enlargement (swelling) of the interdental gingiva, marginal gingiva, or both. As the inflammatory process continues, the marginal gingiva appears rounded with blunted interdental gingiva (Fig. 4-2).

Gingival texture. A reduction in stippling is seen.

Gingival consistency. Consistency varies from soft and spongy (edematous) to firm (fibrotic). In general, the longer the tissues have been affected by the inflammatory process, the more fibrotic the gingiva will appear.

Gingival size. Varying degrees of gingival enlargement occur, depending on the amount of vascular stagnation and tissue proliferation.

Tendency to bleed. Increased tendency to bleed on instrumentation and toothbrushing is noted.

Pain. Chronic gingivitis is usually painless unless complicated by acute exacerbations; it may be painful on instrumentation. Acute inflammation may be superimposed on chronic gingivitis.

Onset. The disease comes on slowly and is of long duration, depending on the length of continued irritation.

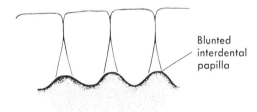

Blunted interdental papilla

FIGURE 4-2. Blunted interdental gingiva characteristic of chronic gingivitis.

Pocket depths. Increased sulcular depth may be present. This is caused by the coronal enlargement of the marginal gingiva because of tissue edema. These pockets are referred to as *gingival pockets* (pseudopockets, relative pockets) (Fig. 4-3, *A*) and should be differentiated from the periodontal pocket, which is characterized by the apical migration of the junctional epithelial attachment to the root surface (Fig. 4-3, *B*). The periodontal pocket is characteristic of periodontitis, not gingivitis.

Exudate. An increased inflammatory but not purulent exudate is characteristic of chronic gingivitis.

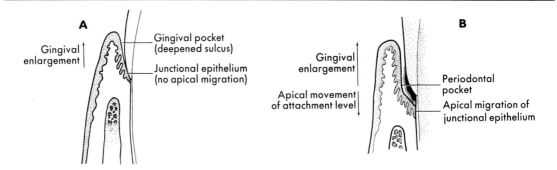

FIGURE 4-3. A, Gingival pocket. B, Periodontal pocket.

Radiographic signs

No radiographic signs are associated with chronic gingivitis because it only affects the soft tissues of the gingiva, which are not recorded on the dental radiograph. If the inflammatory process is allowed to persist, it will gradually invade the deeper periodontal tissues, causing periodontitis. As gingivitis extends to periodontitis, tissue damage that will appear on the radiograph may occur.

Histopathology and pathogenesis

The inflammatory process in gingivitis affects the sulcular and col epithelium along with its underlying connective tissues. The products of the bacterial plaque located adjacent to or within the gingival sulcus or col first cause a disruption of the junctions and intercellular substances that hold the epithelial cells in these areas together. The loosening of the intercellular epithelial junctions provides larger pathways for the microorganisms and their products to follow down into the connective tissues of the gingiva.

In chronic gingivitis the sulcular and col epithelium are characterized by microulcerations and proliferating strands of cells down into the connective tissue. The lamina propria changes associated with this condition include an influx of inflammatory cells, principally plasma cells, lymphocytes, and macrophages. Products of these cells along with the noxious substances

from the plaque microorganisms cause vasodilation, vascular stagnation, collagen fiber destruction, and proliferation of the epithelium. If the inflammation persists over a long period of time, the tissues attempt to repair the damage by forming new collagen fibers. Because of continued irritation in this chronic disease, the repair process is not able to go to completion, and the result is an excess deposition of collagen fibers. This process explains why the gingival tissues become enlarged and leathery (fibrotic) in consistency when the inflammation is present for long periods of time.

The lists on p. 43 correlate the gingival tissue changes that are noted clinically with those noted histologically.

Etiology

The etiology of chronic gingivitis is the accumulation and maturation of bacterial plaque on the teeth, which initiates the inflammatory reaction. Any situation that fosters the accumulation of plaque at the gingival margin is a predisposing factor in chronic gingivitis. Following are typical examples of predisposing factors:

1. Calculus
2. Overhanging gingival margins of restorations
3. Food impaction and retention
4. Frequent exposures to refined sugars or sweets
5. Tooth eruption

Clinically noted changes	Histologically noted changes
Marginal and papillary redness	Vasodilation, engorgement, hyperemia, and proliferation of capillaries
Tendency to bleed on instrumentation in the gingival sulcus and col	Microulceration of the epithelium in the gingival sulcus and col along with engorged capillaries near the surface
Swelling, rounded and blunted contours	Vasostagnation and retention of tissue fluids
Soft, spongy consistency	Vasodilation and destruction of gingival collagen fibers
Reduction in stippling	Edematous condition of the lamina propria
Leathery, firm, and enlarged	Excess deposition of collagen fibers associated with long-standing chronic gingivitis

For further information on local factors refer to Chapter 2.

Nutritional implications

Nutritional deficiencies can affect the way the gingival tissues react to the local irritating factors, but they have never been shown through research to cause gingival inflammation. (See section on nutritional disturbances and deficiencies in Chapter 2.) The consistency of the diet has been shown to have an effect on the development of gingivitis. Soft, retentive foods, especially those consisting of refined sugars, provide oral bacteria the substrate needed for the production of bacterial irritants and plaque. The frequency of sugar exposures is directly related to bacterial growth and plaque formation.

Prognosis

The prognosis of chronic gingivitis depends on the ability of the patient and the dental team to control or eliminate the local etiological factors. If the causative factors are controlled, the gingival tissues will heal and repair themselves because gingivitis is a reversible lesion.

However, if the etiological factors are not controlled the prognosis is not favorable. If the inflammatory process is allowed to persist, it may gradually invade the deeper periodontal tissues, resulting in periodontitis. However, all persistent gingivitis does not become periodontitis.

Treatment

The treatment of chronic gingivitis is aimed at eliminating the local etiological factors to control the agents that initiate the inflammatory process. The gingivitis lesion tries to heal and repair itself, but because of continued local irritation, the healing process is not allowed to go to completion. Treatment of gingivitis is concerned with creating a dentogingival environment that will allow healing to take place.

Treatment consists of eliminating as many of the etiological factors as possible. Typical treatment for a patient with moderate gingivitis is as follows (Fig. 4-4).

1. Diagnosis and assessment of etiological factors
2. Implementation of the following treatment plan and repetition of plan until gingival health is attained
   a. Patient education and instruction in plaque control
   b. Thorough removal of all supragingival and subgingival calculus by scaling the teeth
   c. Removal and provisional replacement of dental restorations and any prosthetic appliances contributing to the gingival disease
   d. Treatment of carious lesions contributing to plaque accumulation
   e. Evaluation of patient's diet with appropriate recommendations for modifications and/or supplementation
   f. Reevaluation of gingival health

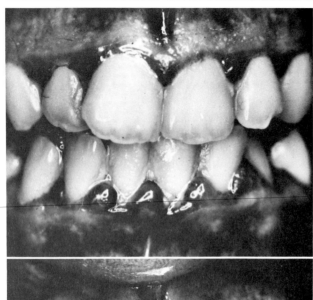

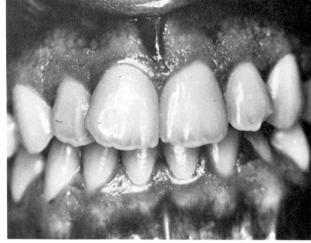

FIGURE 4-4. A, Chronic gingivitis in 25-year-old woman. Note gingival color changes, rounded contours, enlarged size, and accumulations of dental plaque. **B,** Eight weeks following the scaling and root planing procedure. Note the uniform color, tapered contours, and normal size of the gingival tissues.

3. Establishment of recall interval (3 to 6 months) based on patient's cooperation, rate of plaque and calculus accumulations, and tendency for recurrent disease.

Patient education

The success of treatment is directly related to the patient's understanding of the nature and causes of the disease and willingness to perform those oral hygiene procedures necessary to maintain gingival health. The details of im-

plementing an effective plaque control program are described in Chapter 12.

Preventive measures

The prevention of chronic gingivitis involves eliminating the etiological factors before they cause the disease. This program usually involves the following:

1. Maintenance of plaque control consistent with gingival health
2. Effective removal of supragingival and subgingival calculus at intervals frequent

enough to prevent appreciable accumulations

3. Placement of dental and prosthetic restorations with contours compatible with gingival health by avoiding overhanging gingival margins, open interproximal contact points, bulky contours, and partial dentures or any other appliances that impinge on the gingival tissue
4. Intake of a nutritionally adequate diet with reduction of refined sugars
5. Performance of orthodontics when indicated to provide tooth positions that foster good periodontal anatomy and easy plaque control

Chronic gingivitis modified by systemic factors

The etiology of chronic gingivitis can be a combination of local irritating factors such as plaque and calculus, which initiate the inflammatory reaction, and systemic factors, which modify the body's tissue response to the irritation. Following are examples of these conditions:

1. Gingivitis associated with vitamin C deficiency
2. Gingivitis associated with leukemia
3. Gingivitis associated with puberty
4. Gingivitis associated with pregnancy

Gingivitis associated with vitamin C deficiency

Scurvy is a disease in humans that results from a severe vitamin C deficiency. A definite vitamin C deficiency in itself cannot cause gingival inflammation. However, gingivitis caused by local irritants may occur in a patient with a vitamin C deficiency, which tends to exaggerate the gingival inflammatory response. All patients deficient in vitamin C do not have gingivitis; it will only develop if local irritants such as plaque are present.

A severe vitamin C deficiency creates an increased tendency for internal gingival hemorrhage, degeneration of collagen fibers, and edema of the connective tissue. These changes modify and aggravate the response of the gin-

giva to the local irritants. By correcting the vitamin C deficiency, the severity of the gingival inflammation may be reduced, but the gingivitis will still be present until the local irritants are removed.

Clinical characteristics

Gingival color. The gingiva appears to be bluish red.

Gingival contour. Enlargement of the marginal gingiva is seen.

Gingival consistency. The gingiva is soft and friable with a smooth shiny surface. Surface necrosis with pseudomembrane formation may be present.

Tendency to bleed. Tendency to bleed spontaneously or on instrumentation is increased.

Pocket depth. Increased sulcular depth may be present, causing gingival pockets.

In addition to correcting the vitamin C deficiency, treatment also involves complete removal of local irritants.

Gingivitis associated with leukemia

Leukemia is a disease of the blood-forming tissues characterized by the production of excessive numbers of immature white blood cells.

The oral manifestations of leukemia are identical for all forms of the disease, although oral changes are seldom associated with the chronic form of leukemia.

In all forms of leukemia the local irritants such as plaque and calculus initiate the oral changes associated with the inflammatory reaction. If gingivitis does occur in a patient with leukemia, it is caused by the local irritants. The histological changes associated with leukemia modify and aggravate the inflammatory response of the gingiva to the local irritants.

Clinical characteristics

Gingival color. Color is purplish blue because of the stagnation of the blood in the gingival tissues.

Gingival contour. Enlargement of the marginal or interdental gingiva forms tumor-like masses, rounding of the gingival margin, and blunting of the interdental gingiva.

Gingival consistency. The gingiva is moderately firm with a tendency toward friability. It has a shiny surface. Ulceration, necrosis, and pseudomembrane formation may be seen.

Tendency to bleed. Tendency to bleed either spontaneously or on instrumentation is increased.

Pocket depth. Gingival pockets usually form because of the edematous gingival enlargement.

Treatment. Following consultation with the patient's physician to determine appropriate medical precautions, the treatment consists of eliminating all local irritants and their sources.

1. Local irritants are initially eliminated through scaling and polishing of the teeth.
2. Rigid oral hygiene and plaque control procedures are required for the control of all local irritants.
3. Frequent recall visits are necessary to prevent recurrence.

Gingivitis in puberty (Figs. 2-9 and 4-6)

Definition. Inflammation of the gingiva during puberty is also referred to as puberty gingivitis.

Clinical characteristics

Gingival color. The gingiva appears red to bluish red because of increased vascularity within the tissues.

Gingival contour. Enlargement affects both the marginal and the interdental gingiva and is more pronounced on the facial surfaces. Gingival enlargement appears in areas where the local irritants are present.

Gingival consistency. Interdental gingiva appears bulbous and edematous, smooth, and shiny.

Tendency to bleed. Tendency to bleed is increased.

Incidence. Puberty gingivitis affects both males and females.

Extent. If left untreated, gingivitis may become progressively worse and involve the deeper structures of the periodontium.

The inflammatory response to the local irritants is greater than one would expect if adverse hormonal systemic influences were not present. The accentuated response begins at puberty and should subside when the patient is about 17 to 18 years old.

Radiographic signs. No radiographic findings are associated with gingivitis during puberty, since it affects only the soft tissues.

Histopathology and pathogenesis. The histopathological characteristics of gingivitis during puberty are the same as those for chronic gingivitis.

Etiology. Local irritating factors must be present to initiate the gingival changes during puberty. Puberty itself does not cause the inflammatory response. The hormonal changes characteristic of puberty are considered to be responsible for the exaggerated inflammatory response to the local irritants. Therefore the primary etiological factors are the local irritants, and the hormonal changes are secondary or modifying factors.

In addition to plaque, calculus, and inadequate restorative dentistry, common predisposing local factors include malposed and crowded teeth, excessive overbite, orthodontic appliances, mouth breathing, and inadequate diet.

Nutritional implications. The etiological factors of gingivitis in puberty are local and hormonal in nature; therefore nutritional deficiencies are not considered to be direct causative agents. However, poor nutrition in adolescence is common because of poor food selection, voluntary diet restrictions, and fad diets. Nutritional deficiencies can result from these improper eating habits, which in turn may contribute to the exaggerated inflammatory response. In addition, a diet that consists primarily of foods with a soft consistency and retentive sugars can contribute to greater plaque accumulation and subsequent gingivitis.

Prognosis. The gingival enlargement and edema will not disappear automatically at the termination of puberty if local factors are still present. As puberty subsides or ends, the severity of the gingival reaction diminishes. Before the tissues can return to their normal state all local irritants must be completely removed.

If the condition is treated properly and good oral hygiene techniques are used, a healthy gingiva can be maintained. The disease will recur if the local irritants are not kept under control. If the local factors are not eliminated, the condition may progress and cause destruction to the deeper periodontal tissues.

Treatment. Treatment of gingivitis during puberty consists of eliminating all local irritants and their sources.

1. Local irritants are initially eliminated through scaling and polishing of the teeth.
2. Gingivectomy is indicated for severe gingival enlargement.
3. Rigid oral hygiene and plaque control procedures are required for the complete removal of all local irritants.
4. Predisposing factors, such as malposed and crowded teeth, severe overbite, mouth breathing, food impaction, and poor diet, should be corrected.
5. Frequent recall visits are necessary to prevent recurrence.

Patient education. Patients should be informed of the nature and progress of the disease and of their role in helping to control the local irritants.

Plaque control procedures should include toothbrushing technique instruction using a soft, multitufted toothbrush. The sulcular brushing method is recommended. Flossing for interproximal cleaning is also necessary.

If diet is inadequate, nutritional counseling is advised to improve the quality of the patient's diet.

Preventive measures. The major preventive measure for gingivitis during puberty is the elimination of all local irritating factors. Frequent recall visits and repeated instructions in plaque control are necessary to prevent recurrence of the initial disease. Review of dietary factors involved in gingival health and plaque control is also a valuable preventive measure.

Gingivitis in pregnancy (Fig. 4-5)

Definition. Inflammation of the gingiva during pregnancy is also referred to as pregnancy gingivitis.

Clinical characteristics

Gingival color. Color of the gingiva appears bright red to bluish red. This color is related to an increased vascularity within the tissues.

Gingival contour. The inflammatory reaction is more pronounced in the interdental gingiva which appears enlarged (swollen). The marginal gingiva may appear rounded (Fig. 4-5).

Gingival consistency. The interdental and marginal gingiva are edematous in consistency, smooth and shiny in appearance, and friable.

Tendency to bleed. Tendency to bleed on instrumentation is increased.

Extent. The exaggerated gingival response may begin during the second or third months of pregnancy and is the most severe during the second and third trimesters. The gingival inflammation is usually generalized throughout the entire mouth. The inflammatory process may progress into the deeper periodontal tissues and cause damage to these structures.

Pregnancy tumors. Localized areas of the interdental gingiva may become extremely large and form tumorlike growths often referred to as pregnancy tumors. This is not a true tumor. It appears as a mass of bulbous tissue extending from the interdental gingiva. Its color is deep red or magenta, and it has a smooth, shiny surface appearance.

Radiographic signs. No radiographic findings are associated with gingivitis in pregnancy, since it only affects the soft tissues. If the inflammatory condition progresses into the deeper periodontal tissues, damage to these structures may appear on the radiograph.

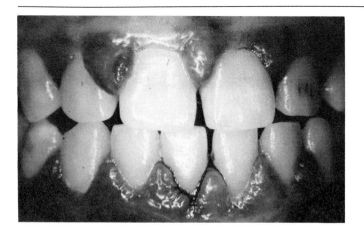

FIGURE 4-5. Gingivitis in a pregnant patient, age 23. Note the enlarged interdental gingiva, the increased tendency to bleed, and the friable texture of the gingiva.

Histopathology and pathogenesis. The histological findings of gingival disease in pregnancy include marked infiltration of inflammatory cells, edema, degeneration of the connective tissue, and hyperplastic epithelium with enlarged rete peg formation. The number of engorged capillaries is also increased.

Etiology. Local irritating factors such as bacterial plaque are primarily responsible for the initiation of gingivitis during pregnancy. Pregnancy in itself does not initiate the inflammatory response and is therefore considered to be a secondary rather than a primary etiologic factor. However, there is a definite increase in the levels of the hormones estrogen and progesterone during pregnancy. The increased severity of gingivitis during pregnancy has been attributed primarily to the increased amounts of progesterone. This hormone has been associated with vasodilation of the gingival blood vessels, circulatory stasis, and increased suseptibility to mechanical irritation. These changes are consistent with the clinical findings of pregnancy gingivitis. It has also been found that there is an increased proportion of the microorganism *Bacteroides melaninogenicus*, subspecies *intermedius* during pregnancy. This is considered an important periodontal pathogen and is associated with increased levels of estradiol and progesterone.

Nutritional implications. The primary etiological factors of gingivitis in pregnancy are local in nature; therefore no nutritional implications are responsible as causative agents.

Prognosis. The gingival inflammation will not disappear automatically at the termination of the pregnancy if the local irritants are still present. The severity of the condition is reduced, but the tissues will not return to their normal healthy state. The gingival enlargement will be reduced in size but not eliminated.

If the condition is treated properly and effective oral hygiene techniques are used, a healthy gingiva can be maintained. The gingival disease will recur if the local irritants are not kept under control.

If the local factors are not eliminated, the condition may progress and cause destruction to the deeper periodontal tissues.

Treatment. Treatment of gingivitis during pregnancy consists of the elimination of all local irritating factors and their sources.

1. Scaling and curettage are indicated for the removal of the local irritants and the inflamed sulcular tissues.
2. Treatment of the tumorlike growth (pregnancy tumor) consists of surgical excision.
3. Rigid plaque control procedures are re-

quired for the elimination and control of all local irritants.

4. Frequent recall visits are necessary to prevent recurrence.

Patient education. Patients should be informed of the nature and progress of the disease and of their role in helping to control the local irritants.

Plaque control procedures include the following:

1 Toothbrushing using a soft, multitufted toothbrush and the sulcular brushing method or roll technique
2. Flossing for interdental cleaning
3. Interdental stimulation following the removal of all calculus if the interdental gingiva remains slightly bulbous

Preventive measures. As a preventive measure all pregnant patients should be seen as early as possible in the pregnancy. Patients should be instructed in plaque control and oral hygiene procedures and in the importance of the control of local irritants. All pregnant patients should be placed on a periodic recall program.

The major preventive measure for gingivitis during pregnancy is the immaculate elimination and control of all local irritants before and during pregnancy.

Other hormonal alterations associated with gingivitis

Oral contraceptives. Oral contraceptives that produce hormonal alterations have been known to exaggerate tissue response to local irritants in a manner similar to pregnancy. This response produces a gingivitis that is usually not as severe.

Gingival changes during menstruation. Preceding or during the menstrual period some patients may exhibit the following gingival symptoms: bleeding, sensitivity to touch or brushing, and edema or slight redness. These changes are usually the exception rather than the rule. If gingival changes do occur during menstruation, they are attributed to the imbalance in sex hormones causing an exaggerated response to local irritation.

Gingivitis associated with mouth breathing

Mouth breathing may be a local factor in the etiology of gingivitis. It may result from a number of factors:

1. Difficulty in nasal respiration caused by nasal passage obstruction from abnormal nasal development, enlarged adenoids, deviated nasal septum, traumatic injury, and growths in the nasal passages
2. Difficulty in nasal respiration caused by an allergy
3. Residual habit formed during childhood in response to tongue and lip habits
4. Certain sleeping positions

The clinical characteristics of mouth breathing may be present in non-mouth breathers when malposed and protruding teeth prevent the normal closure of the lips (incomplete lip closure).

The exact mechanism by which mouth breathing affects the gingiva is not known. It has been suggested that the gingival changes result from the irritation of excessive drying or the continuous wetting and drying of the tissues. Mouth breathing may also accentuate plaque accumulation at the gingival margin, which may be responsible for the inflammatory tissue change.

Clinical characteristics (Fig. 4-6)

Gingival color. Color varies from red to bluish pink.

Gingival contour. Gingival margins are rounded and interdental gingiva is blunted because of the enlargement of the gingiva in the areas exposed to the air. The maxillary anterior region is the area most commonly involved.

Gingival consistency. Diffuse surface shininess is seen in the exposed areas. Gingiva can be firm (fibrotic) or soft and spongy.

Tendency to bleed. Tendency to bleed on instrumentation is increased.

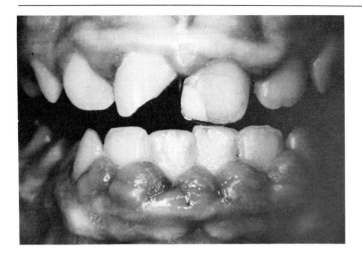

FIGURE 4-6. Gingival enlargement and inflammation in a 13-year-old boy associated with plaque formation, mouth breathing, and puberty.

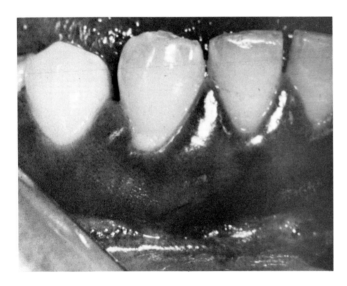

FIGURE 4-7. Diffuse inflammatory gingival changes related to a chewing gum allergy in a 22-year-old woman.

Pocket depth. Gingival pockets are usually present as a result of gingival enlargement.

Treatment

The ideal treatment consists of eliminating or correcting the cause of the mouth breathing.

The following measures may be used:
1. Application of petroleum jelly to the gingiva before retiring
2. Correction of sleeping position
3. Use of a mouth screen during sleep
4. Plaque control if local irritants are present

Allergic gingivitis (Fig. 4-7)

Allergic hypersensitivity involves an abnormal response of the tissues to specific agents. Diverse types and severities of allergic reactions exist. Allergic reactions caused by sensitivity to certain foods or drugs can have oral manifestations as part of a systemic allergic response. The allergic reaction can also be local in na-

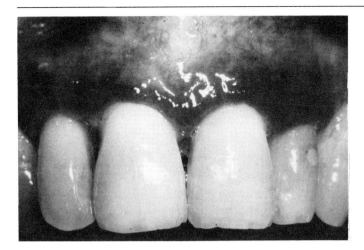

FIGURE 4-8. Desquamative gingivitis in a 40-year-old woman. Note the marginal gingival changes. Histologic diagnosis was lichen planus.

ture, resulting from contact and sensitivity to certain mouthwashes, dentrifrices, and other dental therapeutic agents. The antigen initiates the inflammatory allergic reaction, which is characterized by redness, soreness, gingival necrosis, edema, and ulceration with possible vesicle formation. These symptoms continue as long as the particular agent is used, and the lesions heal on their removal.

Desquamative gingivitis
Definition

Desquamative gingivitis is a rare chronic disease involving the interdental, marginal and attached gingiva. The exact nature of the disease is not fully understood. However, rather than being a specific disease entity, it is now recognized as a clinical manifestation of a variety of diseases, including some dermatoses. These include pemphigus, cicatricial pemphigoid, benign mucous membrane pemphigoid, and lichen planus.

Clinical characteristics (Fig. 4-8)

Chronic desquamative gingivitis occurs in three forms based on the degree of involvement and severity of the clinical characteristics and the advancement of the disease.

Mild
1. Marginal, attached, and interdental gingiva appear reddened.
2. Gingival changes are usually generalized throughout the mouth with the exception of the palatal gingiva.
3. Condition is usually painless.
4. Gingiva will be more severely affected in those areas where local irritants have accumulated—usually the labial surfaces.
5. Alveolar and buccal mucosa may be involved.
6. Periods of exacerbation and spontaneous remission occur.

Moderate
1. Irregular areas of the marginal and attached gingiva appear bright red, smooth, shiny, and soft. A few patches of relatively normal tissue are found among the diseased tissue.
2. Surface epithelium is easily peeled away, exposing the bleeding surface of the underlying connective tissue.
3. Condition is painful.
4. Patients experience a painful burning sensation caused by thermal changes, intake of air, and certain spicy foods and carbonated beverages.

5. Labial surface is usually more severely involved because of local irritants.

Severe

1. Irregular areas on the entire gingiva appear fiery red, smooth, and shiny because of the exposed underlying connective tissue.
2. Gingiva around these denuded areas appears grayish blue.
3. Surface epithelium can be peeled off, exposing red, raw connective tissue.
4. Blisterlike eruptions form and break, exposing the raw, bleeding connective tissue.
5. Lesions are usually confined to the gingiva and occasionally occur in the alveolar mucosa, buccal mucosa, and the hard palate, causing a smooth, shiny appearance.
6. Condition is extremely painful.
7. Patients experience a painful burning sensation caused by thermal changes, air intake, and certain foods and beverages.

Chronic desquamative gingivitis most often affects women, but it is seen occasionally in men. It frequently affects menopausal women, but it may occur any time after puberty.

Although edentulous areas can be affected this seldom occurs.

Inflammation dominates the clinical picture and results from the invasion of bacterial products into the tissues. The inflammatory reaction is a secondary reaction to the initial degenerative disturbance.

Labial surfaces are usually more severely involved because of the accumulation of local irritants.

Radiographic signs

Since the disease only affects the gingival tissues, no radiographic findings are seen. The inflammatory process may progress into the deeper tissues of the periodontium and cause destructive changes that appear on a radiograph. This advanced condition is rare because the patient usually seeks treatment early.

Histopathology and pathogenesis

The histopathologic changes typical of this condition are as follows:

1. Atrophy and thinning of the epithelium
2. Inflammatory infiltrate and retained tissue fluid in the connective tissue
3. Separation of the epithelium from the connective tissue

Etiology

The etiology of chronic desquamative gingivitis is unknown.

The current opinion is that desquamative gingivitis is primarily a degenerative condition of the gingival connective tissue with secondary inflammatory changes. The etiology of the degenerative changes is unknown; however, insufficient gonadal hormones, immunological abnormalities, and nutritional deficiencies have been suggested. The inflammatory changes are related principally to plaque. However, other irritants include hot, spicy foods.

Nutritional implications

Nutritional deficiencies may be a systemic etiological factor or a contributing factor to the disease. Evidence indicates that it may be caused by some inborn errors in metabolism or by a vitamin deficiency. Therapeutic vitamins may be prescribed if indicated after dietary analysis and evaluation.

Prognosis

The prognosis of this disease is difficult to determine because of the unknown etiology. Periods of spontaneous remission and exacerbations can occur and are not necessarily related to treatment. In most cases the pain can be reduced or eliminated through control of the inflammation even though the gingival redness persists.

Treatment

Local treatment. Treatment principally involves removal of local irritants to control the inflammation and avoidance of irritating foods.

A gingivectomy to remove the involved tissues has been suggested as well. While local therapy has helped in some cases, control of the cause of the degenerative changes is more difficult. Local treatment includes the following:

1. Scaling and polishing
2. Instruction in plaque control
3. Topical application of corticosteroids
4. Application of estrogenic hormones in ointment form
5. Protective plastic devices in extremely painful cases and when mastication is difficult

Systemic treatment. Systemic treatment is a supplement to local treatment and is used only as a last resort in very painful cases. Systemic corticosteroid therapy reduces the pain and improves the gingival condition. Caution is indicated when prescribing corticosteroids because side effects can develop after prolonged treatment.

Therapy is continued until improvement occurs and can be terminated without recurrence of the disease.

Because of the unknown etiology, treatment procedures are vague.

Patient education

1. Patients should be informed of the nature and progress of the disease and of their role in helping to control the local irritants.
2. Patients should be discouraged from using oxygenating mouthwashes because they are contraindicated for the condition.
3. Warm water rinses are helpful.
4. Spicy, hot foods, alcohol, and carbonated beverages should be avoided because they irritate the tissues.
5. Patients should eat a well-balanced diet and take vitamin supplements if necessary.
6. Patients should relax and avoid stressful situations.
7. Physical examination may be necessary.

8. Brushing should be done even if painful to eliminate local irritants. A very soft toothbrush should be used. A gentle vibratory motion directing the bristles at the opening of the gingival sulcus is recommended.

Preventive measures

Because the etiology is unknown and ill defined, preventive measures are vague and difficult to identify.

A balanced diet and regular periodic physical and dental checkups are the primary preventive measures. Excellent oral hygiene is also important.

ACUTE CONDITIONS
Acute necrotizing ulcerative gingivitis
Definition

Acute necrotizing ulcerative gingivitis is an acute inflammatory infection of the gingiva. It is also known as Vincent's gingivitis, Vincent's infection, and trench mouth.

Clinical characteristics (Fig. 4-9)

Involvement may be limited to a single tooth or group of teeth or be generalized throughout the mouth. Wide individual variation is seen.

Mild (early stage)
1. Necrosis and ulceration of the tips of the interdental gingiva
2. Gingival bleeding on pressure
3. Possible absence of pain

Advanced (acute stage)
1. Pain (may be severe)
2. Foul metallic taste
3. Foul odor (*fetor ex ore*)
4. Sudden onset
5. Hemorrhage
6. Increased saliva
7. Whitish, graying slough on marginal gingiva—pseudomembrane
8. Involvement of both the labial and the lingual marginal gingiva—red, shiny, and hemorrhagic appearance
9. Attached gingiva rarely affected

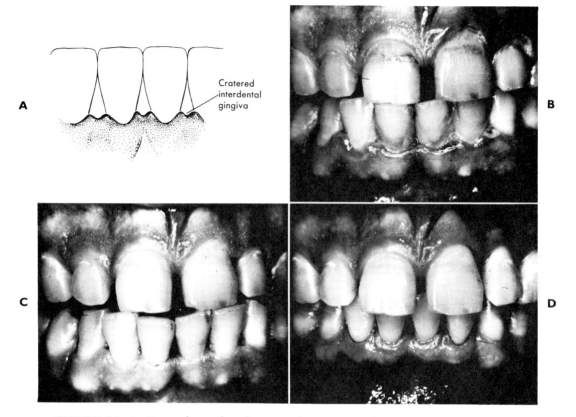

FIGURE 4-9. A, Cratered interdental gingiva characteristic of acute necrotizing ulcerative gingivitis. **B,** Acute necrotizing ulcerative gingivitis. Note the cratered interdental gingiva and the gray-white pseudomembrane. **C,** One month following instructions in plaque control and scaling of the teeth. Note reduction in inflammation but persistence of gingival craters. **D,** Three months following gingivectomies to recontour the cratered gingival contours.

10. Eroded, punched out, and clipped off appearance of interdental gingiva because of ulcerative destruction (Fig. 4-9, A and B)

Severe

1. Swollen and painful regional lymph glands
2. Pharyngeal involvement accompanying the gingival infection (Vincent's angina)
3. Lip and tongue ulcers
4. Progressively destructive process destroying the attached gingiva and the underlying periodontal structures resulting in root exposure and osseous deformities
5. Interdental cratering caused by extensive tissue destruction (Fig. 4-9, A and B)
6. Fever and malaise

Acute necrotizing ulcerative gingivitis is often confused with herpetic gingivostomatitis, a viral condition that will be discussed later. Both diseases may occur simultaneously, but that is rare.

Acute necrotizing ulcerative gingivitis most commonly appears in the acute form, but subacute and chronic forms of the disease have been identified.

Radiographic signs

The gingival changes associated with acute necrotizing ulcerative gingivitis will not appear on radiographs, but with remissions and exacerbations the inflammatory condition may cause destruction of the bony structures. If osseous deformities are present, they will appear radiographically as loss of the lamina dura and/or alveolar bone.

Histopathology and pathogenesis

In general the lesion is characterized histologically by an invasive, nonspecific, acute necrotizing inflammatory condition. The gingival epithelium is destroyed and replaced with a meshwork of fibrin, nonvital epithelial cells, polymorphonuclear leukocytes, and microorganisms. The last comprises the grayish white pseudomembrane seen clinically. The connective tissue is marked by a dense infiltration of inflammatory cells, engorgement of blood vessels, and the presence of spirochetal microorganisms.

Etiology

The exact etiology of acute necrotizing ulcerative gingivitis is not fully established or understood. Numerous factors have been identified, but controversy exists over which factors play primary and contributory roles.

Evidence indicates that the disease occurs as a result of a combination of bacterial, systemic, and psychogenic factors.

The spirochetes *(Borrelia vincentii)* and fusiform bacilli *(Fusobacterium nucleatum)* are markedly increased in number during the disease. However, it has not been established whether the bacteria initiate the disease or are merely secondary factors. Neither of these organisms nor any other has been proved to be the primary etiologic agent of acute necrotizing ulcerative gingivitis. A complex of many microorganisms is more likely involved rather than a single type of organism. Current concepts indicate that the etiology involves a combination of microorganisms and lowered tissue and general body resistance. The latter may be related to nutritional, metabolic, or psychological changes.

Experimentation and reports indicate that the disease is not a communicable infection.

Following are some common local predisposing factors:

1. Poor oral hygiene
2. Calculus
3. Impacted food
4. Excessive smoking and consumption of alcoholic beverages
5. Preexisting gingivitis
6. Periodontal pockets
7. Poor nutrition

It is important to remember that the disease may occur in the absence of any or all of these factors.

The fact that acute necrotizing ulcerative gingivitis may be found in a relatively clean mouth with few local factors gives evidence to support the fact that psychogenic factors are of importance in the etiology. These factors include emotional stress, fatigue, fear, anxiety, and tension.

The most common age group affected is 15 to 25 years old. College students during final exams are greatly affected because of the changes in living styles.

Acute necrotizing ulcerative gingivitis can also be related to systemic disorders and deficiencies. This condition may be brought about by a nutritionally poor diet that results in specific deficiencies such as vitamins C and A and protein. Increased susceptibility to infection can also be present with systemic conditions such as diabetes, leukemia, anemia, and infectious mononucleosis.

Nutritional implications

Acute necrotizing ulcerative gingivitis can often be found in association with vitamin B complex and C deficiencies. Evidence and research seem to indicate that nutritional factors are related to the etiology. Nutritionally deficient diets can contribute to the disease. As a treatment procedure the patient is advised to improve the quality of the diet and to take vitamin supplements if needed after completing a dietary analysis and evaluation session. A soft, bland diet is also recommended during the first week of treatment for patient comfort.

Prognosis

If initial treatment is started in time and follow-up treatment carried through, the gingiva will return to a healthy state with no permanent tissue damage.

If left untreated, acute necrotizing ulcerative gingivitis can lead to progressive destruction of the gingiva and underlying tissues. This destruction can cause permanent damage such as bone loss. Untreated, this disease can also lead to serious systemic conditions.

If preventive measures and follow-up treatment are not established, recurrence is frequent. Repeated attacks can lead to gingival and osseous deformities. Surgical procedures may be needed to correct these deformities.

Treatment

First appointment

1. Patient history is obtained.
2. Clinical symptoms are examined, and a diagnosis is determined. A bacterial smear may be used in conjunction with clinical symptoms for diagnosis. However, the presence of spirochetes and fusiform bacilli is not diagnostic without the accompanying clinical symptoms.
3. Mild, gentle, superficial debridement is performed.
   a. Topical anesthetic may be necessary, depending on patient pain.
   b. Ultrasonic instruments are particularly helpful in performing the debridement.
4. Antibiotics may be prescribed if the patient has an elevated body temperature or cervical lymphadenopathy.

5. Patient is instructed in effective oral hygiene procedures.
6. Other recommendations:
   a. Regular use of chlorhexidine rinses
   b. Reduction or elimination of contributing etiological factors such as fatigue, alcohol consumption, excessive smoking, stress, and poor nutritional habits
   c. Improved dietary habits with a multiple vitamin and mineral supplement prescribed during the recovery phase if necessary
7. The condition, its causes, and its implications should be explained to the patient.

Second appointment (24 to 48 hours after first appointment)

1. At this time marked improvement in the gingival condition should be seen.
2. Supragingival scaling and subgingival debridement are continued. A topical anesthetic may be necessary again, although by this time the pain should have greatly subsided.
3. Use of oral rinses and the elimination of other contributing etiological factors must be discussed and reinforced.
4. Patient should be instructed in toothbrushing techniques using a soft, multitufted toothbrush.

Third appointment (1 week after second appointment)

1. Subgingival scaling and root planing are done.
2. Teeth should be polished.
3. Oral hygiene techniques are reviewed and evaluated.
4. Hydrogen peroxide mouth rinses should be reduced or eliminated to avoid the development of a black hairy tongue.
5. Instruction is given in the use of an interdental stimulator and dental floss.

Fourth appointment (1 week after third appointment)

1. Patient is checked for clinical evidence of a recurrence.

2. Oral hygiene procedures are again reviewed and evaluated.

3. One-month recall appointment is established.

Fifth appointment (I month reevaluation)
(Fig. 4-9, *C*)

1. Patient is checked for clinical symptoms of acute necrotizing ulcerative gingivitis, unphysiological gingival contours, or residual pocket depths.

2. Oral hygiene instruction is reinforced.

3. If periodontal health is restored, a 3-month recall is recommended.

4. If poor gingival architecture or pockets remain, periodontal surgery is recommended (Fig. 4-9, *D*).

Patient education

1. Oral rinses

   a. An effective antimicrobial mouth rinse for this condition is 0.12% chlorhexidine. The patient should rinse with a half ounce of the solution twice each day after brushing.

   b. An alternative is rinsing the mouth with a glassful of equal parts of 3% hydrogen peroxide and warm water. This rinsing consists of forcefully swishing the solution back and forth in the mouth for 3 or 4 minutes. This should be done every 2 or 3 hours for the first 24 to 48 hours. After this time rinses are eliminated or reduced to three times a day, usually after meals. If any undesirable effects appear from the hydrogen peroxide, plain hot water rinses should be used.

   c. Hot water rinses are performed with the same technique except that the patient uses plain hot water to rinse. The water should be as warm as the patient can endure.

2. A soft multitufted toothbrush should be used, and the Bass method of brushing is recommended.

3. Diet is important. A soft, bland diet is usually recommended during the first days of treatment for patient comfort. A vitamin supplement is recommended if the diet has been of a poor quality.

4. Flossing is recommended for interdental cleaning as soon as the acute symptoms have subsided.

5. Interdental stimulation is recommended following the removal of all calculus to aid in the recontouring of the cratered interdental gingiva.

Preventive measures

The patient should be informed of the high rate of recurrence and therefore the need for establishing preventive measures. These would include the following:

1. Proper oral hygiene techniques
2. Nutritious, well-balanced diet
3. Proper rest
4. Avoidance of overstressful situations
5. Avoidance of heavy smoking and alcohol consumption
6. Regular professional prophylaxis—recall

Acute primary herpetic gingivostomatitis
Definition

Acute primary herpetic gingivostomatitis is a viral infection of the oral mucous membranes. It may be confused with acute necrotizing ulcerative gingivitis or desquamative gingivitis. Adequate diagnostic techniques should be used when dealing with these diseases.

Clinical characteristics (Figs. 4-10 and 4-11, *A*)

1. Sudden onset. This self-limiting disease runs its course in 7 to 10 days and usually occurs in preschool children, but may also be seen in adolescents and adults.

2. Painful. Discomfort is felt when eating and brushing.

3. Vesicle formation in oral cavity. Vesicles rupture within 24 hours, forming painful shallow ulcers covered by a grayish

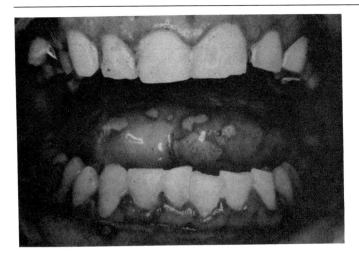

FIGURE 4-10. Acute primary herpetic gingivostomatitis. Note the marginal gingivitis and ulcerative lesions on the tongue and labia mucosa.

membrane. These vesicles can occur anywhere on the oral mucosa—gingiva, labial and buccal mucosa, soft palate, tongue, tonsils, and pharynx. These vesicles vary in size and may appear on the skin and lips (called fever blisters or cold sores).

4. Possible involvement of the gingiva. If the gingiva is involved it will bleed on touch and appear swollen, inflamed, shiny, and edematous.

5. Secondary inflammation. This inflammation is usually the result of invasion of the diseased tissues by the products of the plaque microorganisms. This complicates the disease.

6. Extent. Disease generalized throughout the entire oral mucous membranes, skin, and lips or localized to one or two particular areas.

7. Excessive salivation.

8. Enlargement of cervical lymph glands (cervical lymphadenopathy).

9. Malaise.

10. Fever.

Radiographic signs

No radiographic findings are associated with acute primary herpetic gingivostomatitis, since it only affects the soft tissues of the oral cavity and not the bone.

Histopathology and pathogenesis

Histologically the vesicles are characterized by extracellular and intracellular edema and degeneration of the epithelial cells. The vesicles are located within the layers of epithelium and are a result of fragmentation of the degenerated epithelial cells.

When the vesicles rupture, they leave localized areas of shallow ulceration that are noted histologically by a central zone of acute inflammation, ulceration, and purulent exudate surrounded by an area of engorged blood vessels.

The diagnosis is usually made from information gained in the patient's history and clinical findings.

Etiology

Acute primary herpetic gingivostomatitis is caused by a herpes simplex virus. This disease usually affects infants and children between the ages of 6 months and 10 years of age. It can occur in adults; however, the majority of the adult population have developed an immunity to the disease.

The disease may occur during or immediately after acute infections such as infectious

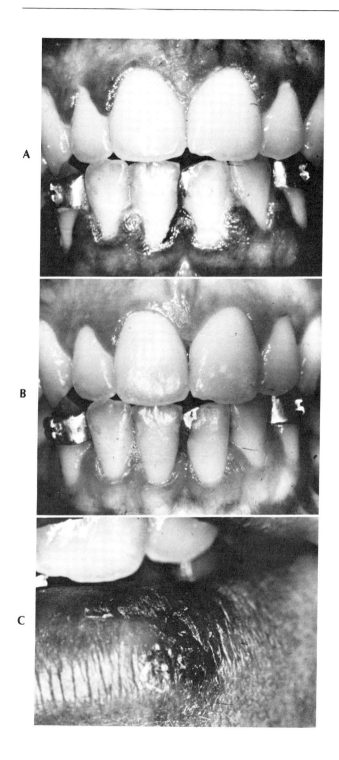

FIGURE 4-11. **A,** Primary acute herpetic gingivostomatitis in 25-year-old woman. **B,** Same patient 10 days following supportive treatment only. Note healing without scarring of tissue. **C,** Same patient 1 year later. Fever blister is a secondary herpetic lesion.

mononucleosis, pneumonia, herpetic infections, and colds. It often manifests itself during periods of lowered resistance, anxiety, and stress, and fatigue. It may occur in the localized form following trauma during dental operative procedures. It is contagious.

Nutritional implications

Nutritional deficiencies do not play a direct role in the etiology of this disease. However, dietary considerations are important in the management of the patient who is experiencing this disease.

Because the ulcers of acute primary herpetic gingivostomatitis are sensitive and painful, foods that are chemically and mechanically irritating as judged by the patient are to be avoided. A diet that is nutritionally adequate and low in retentive sugars is recommended for health of oral tissues. In certain cases dietary supplements in the form of liquid nutritional products are advisable, especially when an inability to chew and swallow food is seen. Dehydration can be a problem with these patients, and therefore copious fluid intake is an important supportive therapy. Currently evidence exists that lysine (an amino acid) therapy provides relief for some patients with herpes simplex infection.

Prognosis

The disease runs its course in 7 to 10 days, and the vesicles and ulcerations heal with no scar formation (Fig. 4-11, *B*). Acute primary herpetic gingivostomatitis is not a recurrent disease because of the formation of antibodies against the virus. However, following the initial infection the individual carries the virus in a latent form in the oral tissues. The virus may be reactivated by any condition that lowers the resistance of the surrounding tissues, resulting in secondary herpetic lesions. The latter are characterized by "fever blisters" on the external surface of the lips and localized ulcerations on the firmly attached oral mucosa (Fig. 4-11, *C*). These lesions need to be differentiated from aphthous lesions (canker sores), which are recurring discrete ulcers usually located on the lining mucosa rather than the masticatory mucosa.

Treatment

1. Diagnosis is established by identifying clinical symptoms and evaluating the patient's history.
2. Mild, gentle superficial debridement of hard and soft deposits is done with ultrasonic instrumentation. Debridement is performed to avoid secondary inflammation caused by the bacterial plaque.
3. Systemic antibiotic therapy is recommended to help control secondary bacterial infection.
4. Topical anesthetic mouthwashes are recommended for temporary relief of pain to facilitate eating.
5. Analgesics can be effective for the relief of pain.
6. Copious fluid intake is recommended to avoid dehydration.
7. Oxygenating mouthwashes are contraindicated because they irritate the tissues.
8. Close observation of the patient every few days until the symptoms disappear is recommended to enable early recognition of complications.
9. Patient should be informed that the disease is contagious.

Patient education

Since the patient's mouth is extremely painful, brushing may become difficult. Consequently, soft and hard deposits accumulate and may become the source of secondary inflammation. Therefore good oral hygiene should be stressed to the patient. Brushing should be done with a soft toothbrush. Rinsing with warm water aids in the cleaning process. Further patient education should include the importance of good nutrition, rest, and the possibility of transferring the condition to others.

Preventive measures

Other than avoiding contact with individuals with the condition, no preventive measure exists for the primary infection of the virus.

Gingivitis in children

Periodontal diseases have been found to exist and progress throughout life. A high incidence of gingivitis has been observed in both the primary and the permanent dentition of children. Many surveys have verified the widespread nature of gingivitis in children. A prevalence of over 80% has been reported.

Chronic marginal gingivitis is the most frequently occurring type of gingival condition in childhood. The clinical characteristics and gingival changes associated with gingivitis in children resemble those of gingivitis in adults. The principal etiological factor in childhood gingivitis is the same as that in adult gingivitis—the local irritation from plaque and local factors that create an environment favorable to the accumulation of local irritants.

Eruption gingivitis

One type of gingival condition, gingivitis associated with eruption, is unique to children. Eruption gingivitis is the name given to the inflammatory changes that may occur around an erupting tooth. It is important to note that tooth eruption in itself does not cause gingival inflammation. The dentogingival environment around an erupting tooth is conducive to the accumulation of soft deposits, and these soft deposits initiate the inflammatory reaction. The clinical characteristics and gingival changes associated with eruption gingivitis resemble those of chronic marginal gingivitis.

Sequelae of gingivitis in children

Although gingivitis is common in children, periodontitis is seen only occasionally. Research and clinical evidence indicate that the damage caused to the supporting structures of the teeth by periodontal disease in childhood and early adult life is irreparable, and the characteristics of periodontal disease in adults have their beginning earlier in life. From 13 years of age onward the proportion of persons with periodontal pockets and alveolar bone loss increases. From epidemiological studies it is clear that the prevalence of destructive disease follows a linear progression from adolescence to old age. This fact probably reflects the cumulative nature of the disease as opposed to the diminishing resistance of older people.

The two forms of periodontitis seen in children are prepubertal periodontitis, which affects the primary dentition, and juvenile periodontitis (periodontosis), which may affect the entire permanent dentition or more commonly the first molars and the incisors in adolescents and young adults. Refer to Chapter 7 for further discussions of these conditions.

SUGGESTED READINGS

Carranza F: Glickman's clinical periodontology, ed 5, Philadelphia, 1979, WB Saunders Co, pp 354-373.

Kornman KS, and Loesche WJ: The subgingival microbial flora during pregnancy, J Periodont Res 15:111-122, 1980.

Nisengard RJ: Role of immunology in periodontal disease, J Periodontol 48:505, 1977.

CHAPTER 5
Gingival Enlargement

Gingival enlargement may be associated with the following:
1. Bacterial plaque–induced inflammation
2. Bacterial plaque and the hormonal changes of
   a. Puberty
   b. Pregnancy
3. Blood dyscrasias
4. Medications
   a. Phenytoin
   b. Cyclosporine
   c. Nifedipine
   d. Diltiazem
5. Familial characteristics
6. Mouth breathing
7. Neoplasias

Gingival enlargement can be the result of inflammatory or noninflammatory changes or a combination. In inflammatory gingival enlargement the increase in gingival size results from the infiltration of the connective tissues by fluid and cells of inflammatory exudate (Fig. 5-1, *A* and *B*). The initial enlargement is primarily the result of a stagnation of blood and other tissue fluids and cells in the connective tissue of the gingiva. As the process becomes chronic, the amount of collagen fibers in the gingiva increases, which also results in tissue enlargement. The inflammatory gingival overgrowth in a patient can be exaggerated by other conditions such as puberty, pregnancy, a habit of mouth breathing, certain blood dyscrasias, and medications such as phenytoin, cyclosporine, nifedipine, and diltiazem. See Chapter 4 and Figs. 4-5 and 4-6 for details. Noninflammatory gingival enlargement is most commonly related to the use of medications, familial characteristics, or neoplastic changes. However, with drug-induced and familial gingival enlargements in which the tissue overgrowth is primarily related to noninflammatory hyperplasia, the condition may be aggravated by plaque and associated inflammation.

GINGIVAL ENLARGEMENT ASSOCIATED WITH MEDICATIONS
Phenytoin
Definition

Enlargement of the gingiva occurs in approximately 50% of the patients treated with the anticonvulsant drug phenytoin (Dilantin, Epanutin).

Clinical characteristics (Fig. 5-2)

1. Generalized enlargement of the marginal and interdental gingiva is seen. This coronal enlargement of the gingiva causes an increase in sulcular depth without apical migration of the junctional epithelium.
2. Enlargement is more pronounced in the interdental gingiva areas.
3. Tissue enlargement may progress to the point that the tissue obscures the teeth and may interfere with occlusion.
4. Enlarged tissue appears firm, fibrotic, pale pink, and resilient, has little tendency to bleed, and has a lobed surface appearance.
5. Enlargement is usually generalized throughout the mouth and appears more pronounced in the anterior area.

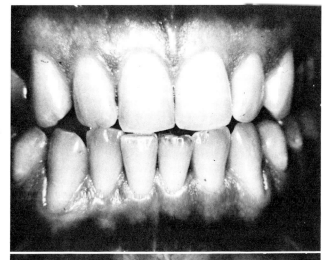

A

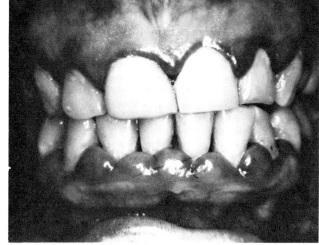

B

FIGURE 5-1. A, Normal gingival size and tapered contours. **B,** Inflammatory gingival enlargement. Note the swollen and rounded gingival contours.

6. Local irritants, if present, may complicate the reaction caused by the drug, resulting in inflammation.
7. If inflammation is present, it changes the clinical picture as follows:
   a. Inflammation increases the size of the already enlarged hyperplastic tissue.
   b. Tissue appears red or bluish red.
   c. Bleeding tendency increases.
   d. Lobed surface appearance is lost.
8. Enlargement affects areas in which teeth are present and rarely affects edentulous spaces.

9. Enlargement occurs more frequently in younger patients receiving the medication.

Radiographic signs

If phenytoin gingival enlargement is uncomplicated by an inflammatory reaction caused by local irritants, no specific radiographic findings characteristic of this condition will be seen because only the soft tissues are affected.

If an underlying periodontitis is present, radiographic findings indicate the loss of the alveolar bone.

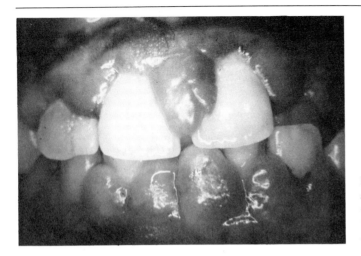

FIGURE 5-2. Gingival enlargement in a 21-year-old woman being treated with the anticonvulsant drug phenytoin. Note that the condition affects primarily the interdental gingiva.

Histopathology and pathogenesis

Hyperplasia is an increase in the size of an organ or its part caused by an increase in the number of cellular elements. Histologically, phenytoin gingival enlargement is a hyperplastic reaction of the connective and epithelial tissues.

The enlargement is predominantly related to an increase in the number of collagen fibers, but the number of fibroblasts, inflammatory cells, and epithelial cells also increases. The exact mechanism of how the drug stimulates the hyperplasia is not known.

This gingival enlargement is not *hypertrophy*, which indicates an increase in the size rather than the number of cells.

Etiology

The tissue enlargement is initially and primarily a hyperplastic reaction to the anticonvulsant drug phenytoin.

The enlarged tissue creates a dentogingival environment that favors the accumulation of bacterial plaque and other soft deposits. The enlarged tissue also interferes with proper oral hygiene techniques. These local factors cause an inflammatory tissue reaction. Therefore phenytoin gingival enlargement can be attributed to the use of phenytoin alone or in con-

junction with local irritants. The combined type is the most common. This is an important concept in relationship to treatment, and the clinical characteristics should be distinguished as to their specific etiology.

Phenytoin hyperplasia may occur in patients whose mouths are free of local irritants, and it may not occur in some patients whose mouths have abundant local irritants.

Nutritional implications

At this time no evidence exists for any nutritional involvement with this condition. Nutritional deficiencies can affect the way the gingival tissues react to the local irritating factors, and therefore good dietary habits are supportive in the health and repair of oral tissues.

Prognosis

If the drug is discontinued, the enlargement usually subsides.

If the condition is not complicated by inflammation and the tissue is surgically removed, recurrence is common with continued use of the drug.

If the condition is combined with inflammation, the prognosis depends on the success of preventive measures for control of local factors. Local treatment is effective, but enlargement can occur solely as a result of using the phenytoin.

Treatment

The treatment of phenytoin gingival hyperplasia is based on its specific etiology.

Phenytoin gingival enlargement not complicated by inflammation caused by local irritants

1. Discontinuing the phenytoin is the only method of eliminating the condition and any possibility of recurrence. If the drug is discontinued, the enlargement usually subsides after 1 or 2 months.
2. Although phenytoin is the drug of choice for treatment of epilepsy, occasionally an alternate drug can be prescribed.
3. If the phenytoin cannot be discontinued, a gingivoplasty is indicated for removal of the extensively enlarged tissue.

Phenytoin gingival enlargement complicated by inflammation caused by local irritants

1. Rigid plaque control should be practiced by the patient to eliminate local factors.
2. All sources of local irritation should be eliminated.
3. Gingivectomy or gingivoplasty should be performed when extensive tissue enlargement is present to recreate a more hygienic dentogingival environment.

Recurrence of the condition can be kept under control by regular periodic scaling and curettage and rigorous plaque control by the patient. These two procedures prevent only the enlargement due to the inflammatory process. They will not prevent the enlargement caused by the phenytoin itself.

Patient education

Patients should be informed of the nature and progress of the disease and of their role in helping to control the local irritants.

Rigorous plaque control procedures include the following:

1. Brushing using the Bass method is recommended, although the enlargement may prevent any established method from being properly used.
2. Dental floss should be used if the enlargement does not interfere with proper utilization.
3. Interdental cleaners and stimulation should be used.
4. Oral irrigating devices have been helpful in cases of extreme enlargement.

Preventive measures

Phenytoin gingival enlargement uncomplicated by inflammation. The only preventive measure is to discontinue the use of phenytoin, changing if necessary to another anticonvulsant drug.

Phenytoin gingival enlargement complicated by inflammation caused by local irritants

1. The use of phenytoin should be discontinued or another anticonvulsant drug should be used to prevent enlargement caused by phenytoin.
2. Rigorous plaque control should be practiced by the patient to eliminate local irritants.
3. All local irritants should be eliminated.
4. Periodic scaling and curettage should be performed.

Cyclosporine

Cyclosporine is an immunosuppressive drug used to help prevent organ transplant rejection and to treat Type I diabetes mellitus and other autoimmune disorders. Gingival hyperplasia is found in approximately one third of the adults taking the drug and more frequently in children. The initial enlargement usually begins in the interdental gingiva, is more common on the labial than the lingual surfaces of the teeth, and is more common in the anterior than the posterior segments of the dentition. The tissue response is more severe when local irritating factors such as plaque and calculus are present. The gingival enlargement is usually reversible if the cyclosporine therapy is discontinued.

The gingival enlargement can be minimized

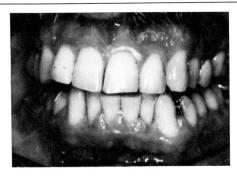

FIGURE 5-3. Gingival enlargement associated with nifedipine (Procardia) and plaque in a 55-year-old man.

during the early phases of the therapy with meticulous plaque control and regular prophylactic measures. Surgical procedures can be used to treat the gingival enlargement, but the incidence of recurrence is not known.

Nifedipine (Procardia) and diltiazem (Cardizem)

Nifedipine and diltiazem are calcium-blocking drugs used to treat angina pectoris, a heart condition. The gingival enlargements are side effects of the medications and are similar to the hyperplastic changes seen with phenytoin therapy (Fig. 5-3).

FAMILIAL (HEREDITARY) GINGIVAL ENLARGEMENT
Definition

Familial or hereditary gingival enlargement is a rare hyperplastic disease with unknown etiological factors resulting in gingival enlargement. It is also commonly referred to as idiopathic gingival hyperplasia.

Clinical characteristics (Fig. 5-4)
1. Attached gingiva, marginal gingiva, and interdental gingiva are enlarged. This increase in gingival size causes an increase in sulcular depth. This condition is referred to as a gingival pocket or pseudo-pocket and is caused by the coronal enlargement of the gingiva.
2. Enlargement usually affects both the facial and lingual surfaces of both arches, but it may be limited to just one arch.
3. Enlarged tissues appear pink, firm, resilient, bulbous, and fibrotic and have no tendency to bleed.
4. Enlarged hyperplastic tissue may progress to the point that the tissue obscures the teeth and may interfere with occlusion.
5. Local irritants can cause inflammation, which complicates the reaction and changes the clinical picture as follows:
   a. Size of the already enlarged hyperplastic tissue is increased.
   b. Tissues appear red or bluish red.
   c. Bleeding tendency increases.

Radiographic signs

If familial gingival enlargement is uncomplicated by an inflammatory reaction, no specific radiographic findings characteristic of this condition are seen, because generally only the soft tissues are affected.

If an underlying periodontitis is present, radiographic findings indicate the loss of the alveolar bone.

Histopathology and pathogenesis

Histologically, familial gingival enlargement is a hyperplastic reaction of the connective and epithelial tissues. The amount of collagen fibers increases and the surface epithelium thickens.

Etiology

The etiology of this hyperplastic condition is unknown, although several theories have been used to explain the reaction.

A major assumption is that an inherited constitutional factor plays a major etiological role. This assumption is based on the fact of multiple occurrences in the same family.

Local irritating factors are complicating etiological factors that accentuate the preexisting

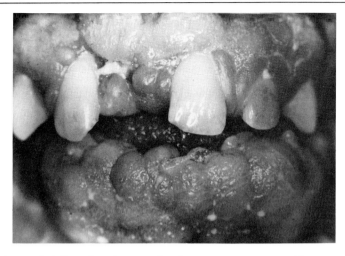

FIGURE 5-4. Familial (hereditary) gingival enlargement in 18-year-old man. Note that the marginal and attached gingiva as well as the interdental gingiva are all affected.

hyperplasia with an inflammatory response. The enlarged tissue creates a favorable environment for the accumulation of plaque and other deposits.

Nutritional implications

At this time no evidence exists of any nutritional involvement with this condition.

Prognosis

On surgical removal the short-term prognosis is favorable; however, on a long-term basis the enlargement will most likely recur. Recurrence may be minimized by complete elimination of all local factors.

Treatment

The treatment consists of surgical removal (gingivectomy) of the excessive enlarged tissue and elimination of the local irritating factors by plaque control and scaling.

Recurrence of the condition can be kept under control by regular periodic scaling and curettage and rigorous plaque control.

These two procedures prevent only the enlargement caused by the inflammatory process.

They will not prevent the portion of the enlargement created by the familial etiological factor.

Patient education

Patients should be informed of the nature and progress of the disease and of their role in helping to control the local irritants.

Plaque control includes the following:
1. Brushing using the Bass method is recommended, although the enlargement may prevent any established method from being properly used.
2. Flossing should be performed if the enlargement does not interfere with its proper utilization.
3. Interdental cleaners and stimulators should be used when possible.
4. Oral irrigating devices have been helpful in cases of extreme enlargement.

Preventive measures

Since the etiology is unknown, no measures are known at this time to prevent the hyperplastic enlargement. If the disease is complicated by an inflammatory reaction, the inflammatory

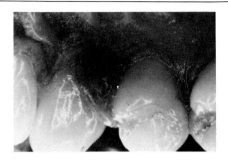

FIGURE 5-5. Fibroma in a 21-year-old woman.

process can be prevented by the elimination of all local irritating factors, a rigorous plaque control program, and periodic scaling and curettage.

NEOPLASTIC GINGIVAL ENLARGEMENT

Only a small proportion of gingival enlargements are related to neoplasms. Common ex-amples are fibromas (Fig. 5-5), papillomas, and mixed tumors (salivary gland type). A discrete gingival enlargement is sometimes referred to as an epulis.

SUGGESTED READINGS

Baer PN, and Morris ML: Textbook of periodontics, Philadelphia, 1977, JB Lippincott Co, pp 318-322.

Carranza F: Glickman's clinical periodontology, ed 5, Philadelphia, 1979, WB Saunders Co, pp 106-134.

Daley TD, Wysocki GP: Cyclosporine therapy. Its significance to the periodontist, J Periodontol 55:708-712, 1984.

Lucas RM, Howell LP, Wall BA, Nifedipine-induced gingival hyperplasia—A histochemical and ultrastructural study, J Periodontol 56:211-215, 1985.

Seymour RA, and Heasman PA: Drugs and the periodontium, J Clin Periodontol 15:1-16, 1988.

Strahan JD, and Waite IM: Color atlas of periodontology, Chicago, 1979, Year Book Medical Publishers, Inc, pp 30-32.

CHAPTER 6
Periodontitis

DEFINITION

Periodontitis is a disease in which the gingiva as well as portions of the periodontal ligament, cementum, and alveolar bone are affected by the inflammatory process. The inflammation begins in the gingiva and subsequently invades the deeper supporting structures. Periodontitis is characterized by gingival inflammation, periodontal pocket formation, destruction of the periodontal ligament and alveolar bone, and gradual loosening of the teeth. The incidence of periodontitis is approximately one in four adults. The incidence of periodontal disease with pocket formation increases gradually with age, being approximately 1% at 10 years of age, 10% at 20 years of age, 20% at 35 years of age, and 40% at 50 years of age. Epidemiological studies also show the following:

1. In general, males have a higher incidence and severity of periodontal disease than females.
2. Blacks have more severe periodontal disease than whites.
3. Periodontal disease is inversely related to increasing levels of education and income.

Periodontitis occurs in different forms and has been classified by Page and Schroeder as follows:

1. Prepubertal periodontitis
2. Juvenile periodontitis
3. Rapidly progressive periodontitis
4. Adult periodontitis

Prepubertal periodontitis, juvenile periodontitis, and rapidly progressive periodontitis are aggressive forms that affect individuals at relatively young ages and have been grouped under the term early onset periodontitis. A description of these conditions is found in Chapter 7. The most common type of the disease is adult periodontitis, which is the subject of this chapter.

CLINICAL CHARACTERISTICS (Fig. 6-1)

The gingiva is usually chronically inflamed. However, its external appearance may vary according to the length of time the disease has been present and to the individual tissue response. In general, with the exception of extremely advanced situations, the longer the tissues have been affected by the inflammatory process, the less red and more leathery the gingiva appear. Typically in moderately advanced periodontitis, the following clinical characteristics are present:

Gingival color

Varying degrees of bluish-red are seen.

Gingival consistency

Consistency varies from soft and boggy (edematous) to firm (fibrotic).

Gingival texture

Stippling is decreased.

Gingival contour

The marginal gingiva is rounded, and the interdental gingiva is blunted.

Gingival size

The gingiva is slightly enlarged.

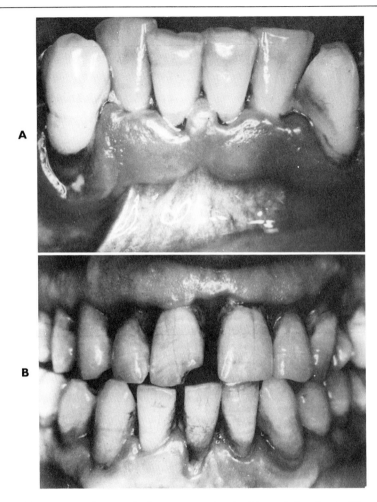

FIGURE 6-1. **A,** Typical gingival changes associated with periodontitis in 50-year-old man: rounded marginal gingiva, blunted interdental gingiva, reduced stippling, fibrotic gingival enlargement, recession, and pocket formation. **B,** Advanced periodontitis in 55-year-old man.

Gingival position

Level of the gingival attachment to the tooth (junctional epithelium) will be at least 3 to 4 mm apical to the cementoenamel junction.

Tendency to bleed

Usually sulcular bleeding on instrumentation is seen.

Probing depths

Increased probing depths are found—usually greater than 2 mm facially and lingually and greater than 3 mm interdentally. Even though the gingiva may appear pink and firm, if deep periodontal pockets are found, periodontitis is usually present.

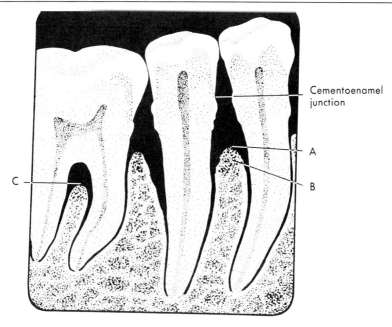

FIGURE 6-2. Radiographic changes consistent with periodontitis. *A*, Crest of alveolar bone more than 2 to 3 mm apical to the cementoenamel junction. *B*, Indistinct crestal bone density. *C*, Radiolucency in furcation areas.

Exudate

Purulent exudate can often but not always be expressed from the pocket with pressure.

Tooth surface

The tooth surface is rough, and calculus is usually present.

Tooth mobility

Mobility varies from none to a moderate increase.

RADIOGRAPHIC SIGNS

Dental radiographs can be of value in determining the extent of periodontal tissue destruction. However, periodontitis *cannot* be diagnosed from a radiographic analysis alone, primarily because soft tissue changes are not recorded on the dental radiograph. The radicular alveolar bone is also not accurately depicted. The following radiographic characteristics are indicative of alveolar bone changes that are consistent with the presence of periodontitis. However, pocket formation and/or changes in the periodontal attachment levels involve soft tissues and must be verified by a clinical examination with a periodontal probe (Figs. 6-2 and 6-3).

1. Crest of the interdental alveolar bone is more than 2 to 3 mm apical to the cementoenamel junction, indicating alveolar bone loss (Figs. 6-2 and 6-3, *B*).
2. Crest of the interdental alveolar bone may appear fuzzy, and the crestal lamina dura is not well defined (Fig. 6-3, *B*).
3. Bifurcation and trifurcation areas between the molar roots may have radiolucencies indicating interradicular bone loss (Figs. 6-2 and 6-3, *C*, *D*, and *E*).

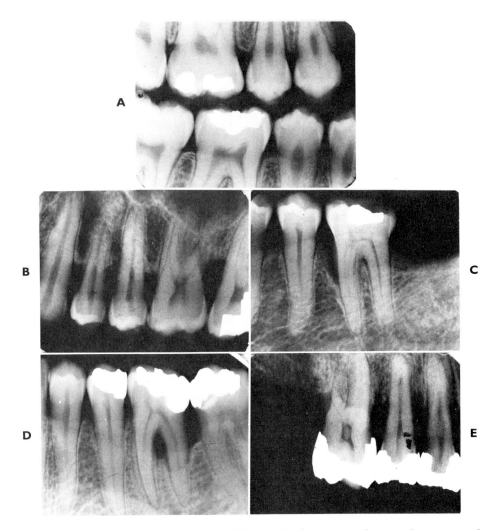

FIGURE 6-3. A, Radiographic image of healthy alveolar bone. Note the smooth contour and radiopaque density (crestal lamina dura) of the crestal portions of the interdental bone and the close proximity between the height of the interdental bone and the cementoenamel junctions. **B,** Radiographic image consistent with periodontitis. Note the uneven contours and the lack of a well-defined crestal lamina dura and the increased distance between the height of the bone and the cementoenamel junctions. **C,** Angular bone contour and early bifurcation involvement. Note the angular radiolucent area on the mesial surface of the molar and the small radiolucency in the bifurcation area. **D,** Definite bifurcation involvement on the first molar and a decrease in the density of the crestal interproximal bone. **E,** Decrease in the density of the interdental bone suggesting bone resorption activity.

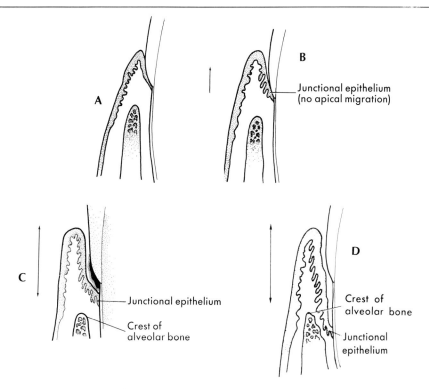

FIGURE 6-4. Types of pockets. **A,** Healthy gingival sulcus. **B,** Gingival pocket—gingival enlargement only (*note arrow*). **C,** Suprabony periodontal pocket—gingival enlargement, apical migration of junctional epithelium (*note arrows*). Deepest portion of the pocket is coronal to the crest of the alveolar bone. **D,** Infrabony periodontal pocket—gingival enlargement, apical migration of junctional epithelium. Deepest portion of the pocket is apical to the crest of the alveolar bone.

4. Density of the interdental bone is decreased (Fig. 6-3, *C*, and *E*).
5. Horizontal and angular patterns of the bone resorption may be noted (Figs. 6-8, *B* and 6-10 *B*).

HISTOPATHOLOGY AND PATHOGENESIS

Periodontitis begins as gingivitis (Fig. 6-4, *B*), and if the inflammatory process is allowed to persist, it will in most but not all patients gradually invade the deeper periodontal tissues. The inflammatory process carries with it the potential to stimulate the resorption of the periodontal tissues and the formation of periodontal pockets.

Periodontal pocket formation

A periodontal pocket is a gingival sulcus that has been deepened by apical migration of the junctional epithelium and destruction of the periodontal ligament and alveolar bone. Gingival enlargement may also contribute to the increased depth (Fig. 6-4, *C*).

While the exact mechanisms of pocket formation are not completely understood, two leading periodontal pathologists, Page and Schroeder, have classified the stages of pathogenesis as follows:

1. *Initial lesion:* Characteristics of the initial lesion are vasculitis of the blood vessels deep to the junctional epithelium, increased flow of gingival fluid, movement

of leukocytes into the junctional epithelium and the gingival sulcus, extracellular serum proteins, alterations of the coronal aspects of the junctional epithelium, and loss of collagen fibers around the gingival blood vessel.

2. *Early lesion:* The early lesion is noted by exaggeration of the initial lesion characteristics, the presence of lymphoid cells beneath the junctional epithelium where the acute inflammation is concentrated, fibroblast alterations, more destruction of the gingival collagen fibers, and early proliferation of the basal cells of the junctional epithelium.

3. *Established lesion:* With an established lesion the acute inflammation manifestations persist; plasma cells predominate; immunoglobulins accumulate extravascularly; destruction of collagen fibers continues; a proliferation, apical migration, and lateral extension of the junctional epithelium is seen; and early periodontal pocket formation is possible, but no appreciable bone destruction occurs.

4. *Advanced lesion:* The advanced lesion is typical of periodontitis and is characterized by continuation of the established lesion features, spread of the lesion into the alveolar bone and periodontal ligament resulting in bone destruction, loss of collagen fibers adjacent to the pocket epithelium, fibrosis in the more peripheral areas, the presence of altered plasma cells, periodontal pocket formation, periods of exacerbation and periods of very little pathologic activity, conversion of bone marrow into fibrous connective tissue, and generalized evidence of inflammatory and immunopathological tissue reactions.

In summary:

1. Gingivitis is initiated by the invasion of the dental plaque bacteria and their products through the junctional and sulcular epitheliums (Fig. 6-5).

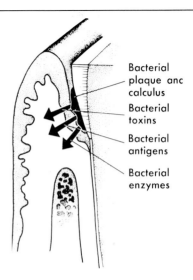

Bacterial plaque anc calculus

Bacterial toxins

Bacterial antigens

Bacterial enzymes

FIGURE 6-5. Products of dental plaque pass through the sulcular epithelium and stimulate the inflammation.

2. Vascular stagnation, retained tissue fluids, and eventual fibrosis of the gingiva result in increased pocket depth by causing gingival enlargement. If this occurs in the absence of apical migration of the junctional epithelium, it is called a *gingival pocket* (Fig. 6-4, *B*), but it can also contribute to the depth of a *periodontal pocket* (Fig. 6-4, *C*).

3. The inflammatory process in the gingiva also stimulates apical proliferation of the epithelial cells that make up the junctional epithelium and sulcular epithelium (Fig. 6-6, *A*).

4. In addition, the inflammatory process is responsible for the degeneration of the gingival fibers, which makes it easier for the proliferating epithelium to move apically along the root surface. As the epithelium migrates apically, the more coronally positioned portions of the junctional epithelium separate from the tooth surface, thereby creating a deepened gingival sulcus (Fig. 6-6, *B*).

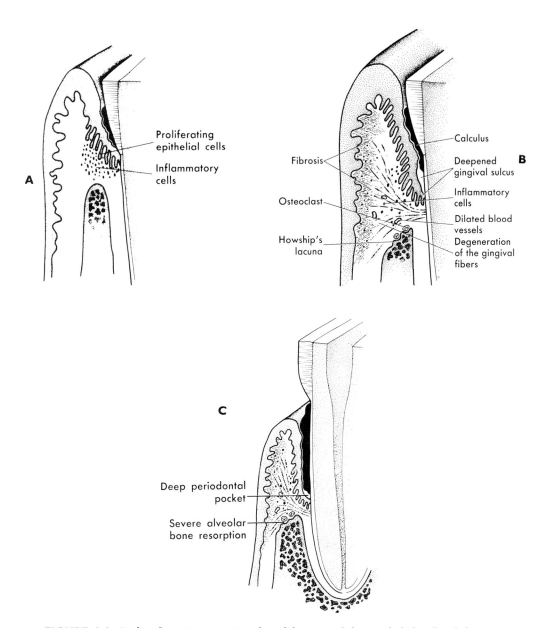

FIGURE 6-6. Pocket formation. **A,** Apical proliferation of the epithelial cells of the junctional epithelium attachment and sulcular epithelium. **B,** Apical movement of the junctional epithelium (deepened gingival sulcus); degeneration of the gingival fibers; osteoclastic bone resorption; fibrosis. **C,** Advanced periodontitis.

5. The inflammatory process also stimulates resorption of the alveolar bone and periodontal ligament fibers just apical to the gingival fibers and removes another barrier to apical migration of the junctional epithelium and pocket formation (Fig. 6-6, *B*).

6. With the formation of pockets periodontal inflammatory disease becomes self-perpetuating in that the principal etiological factor, plaque, can now form in the more anaerobic pocket environment, which encourages the growth of periodontal pathological organisms and is less accessible to removal by the patient. If this sequence of events is allowed to persist over an extended period of time, the chronic infection can cause severe destruction of the periodontium and loss of the teeth (Fig. 6-6, *C*). Current research indicates that there are probably periods of active bone resorption followed by times of inactivity in which periodontal pockets may be present but do not result in further attachment loss. Thus peri-

odontitis is now considered to be a disease in which there are periods of exacerbation (progressing loss of attachment) and remission (minimal or no loss of attachment) rather than linearly progressive as previously thought. The rationale for pocket reduction as part of periodontal therapy is to create a dentogingival environment less likely to accumulate subgingival plaque and more conducive to effective plaque removal by the patient.

Types of periodontal pockets

The two types of periodontal pockets (which does not include gingival pockets) based on the relationship of the junctional epithelium to the crest of the adjacent alveolar bone are suprabony periodontal pockets and infrabony periodontal pockets.

In a suprabony periodontal pocket (Fig. 6-4, *C*) the coronal level of the junctional epithelium (bottom of pocket) is coronal to the crest of the alveolar bone. In an infrabony periodontal pocket (Fig. 6-4, *D*) the coronal level of the

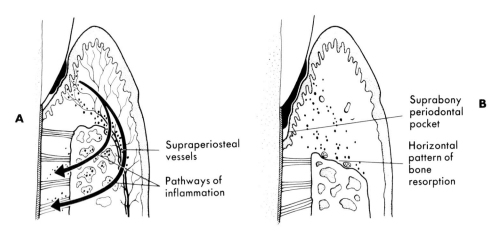

FIGURE 6-7. A, Pathways the inflammatory process usually takes along the supraperiosteal neurovascular bundle from the gingiva to the supporting periodontal tissues on the facial and lingual surfaces of the teeth. **B,** Horizontal pattern of bone resorption and a suprabony periodontal pocket are the usual result when the inflammation follows the pathway illustrated in **A.**

junctional epithelium (bottom of pocket) is apical to the crest of the alveolar bone.

Patterns of alveolar bone and periodontal ligament destruction

The types of pockets that form and the patterns of tissue destruction that occur may depend on the pathway the inflammatory process takes as it spreads from the gingiva to the underlying supporting structures. The pathway of least resistance is usually taken and is most commonly

the connective tissue sheath that surrounds the neurovascular bundles. On the facial and lingual surfaces of the teeth the principal neurovascular bundles are located in the periosteum on the outer surface of the bone (Fig. 6-7, A). In the interproximal bone the vessels and nerves are located within the cancellous portion of the bone approximately midway between the adjacent teeth (Fig. 6-8, A). When the loose connective tissue sheaths that surround these bundles are followed, the inflam-

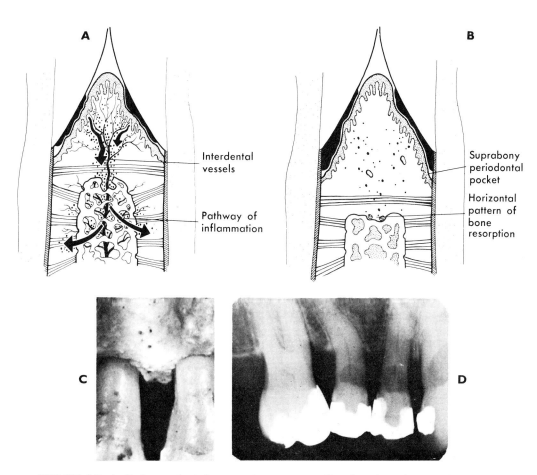

FIGURE 6-8. A, Pathways the inflammatory process usually takes along the interdental neurovascular bundle from the gingiva to the supporting periodontal tissues in the interdental areas. **B,** Horizontal pattern of bone resorption and suprabony periodontal pockets are the usual result when the inflammation follows the pathways illustrated in **A. C,** Horizontal pattern of bone resorption. **D,** Radiograph illustrating a horizontal pattern of bone loss.

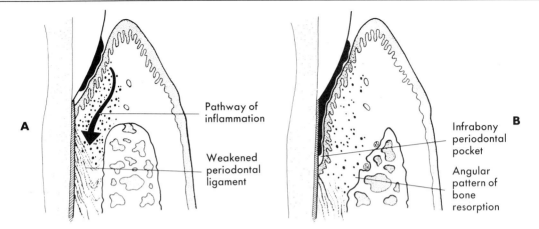

FIGURE 6-9. A, On the facial or lingual aspects of teeth the pathway may be directly into the periodontal ligament space when it has been weakened by excessive occlusal forces. **B,** Angular pattern of bone resorption and infrabony periodontal pockets are the result of the inflammatory process following the pathway directly into the periodontal ligament space.

matory process invades and destroys the supporting alveolar bone first and then spreads laterally to the alveolar bone proper and the periodontal ligament (Figs. 6-7, *A,* and 6-8, *B*). This results in suprabony periodontal pockets and horizontal patterns of bone loss (Figs. 6-7, *B,* and 6-8, *B* to *D*).

Generally the alveolar crestal periodontal ligament fibers create an effective barrier to the spreading inflammation. This is another reason why the supporting alveolar bone is invaded before the periodontal ligament. However, in certain circumstances and in occlusal trauma particularly, the crestal periodontal ligament fibers are weakened and the pathway of least resistance is sometimes modified to follow directly into the periodontal ligament space (Figs. 6-9, *A,* and 6-10, *A*). This results in resorption of the principal fibers and alveolar bone proper before the supporting bone, thereby separating the most coronal portion of the supporting alveolar bone from the periodontal ligament and tooth (Figs. 6-9, *B,* and 6-10, *B*). This bone resorption pattern is angular or vertical, and the pockets are of the infrabony type (Figs. 6-9, *B,* and 6-10, *B* to *D*).

Mechanisms of periodontal tissue destruction

Many studies have been done and several mechanisms have been suggested, but a definitive explanation of how bone is destroyed in inflammatory periodontal disease has not been given.

Osteoclasts and mononuclear phagocytes are increased in the periodontal tissues during inflammatory periodontal disease. Both of these cells are capable of resorbing bone by first removing the minerals and then digesting the exposed collagen. The following factors have been shown to stimulate an increase in osteoclasts:

1. Production of an osteoclast-activating factor from leukocytes stimulated by antigens from dental plaque
2. Increased vascularity associated with inflammation
3. Endotoxin from the microorganism *Bacteriodes melaninogenicus*

Other factors related to bone resorption are parathyroid gland extract, tumor fragments, heparin, prostaglandins, collagenase, hyaluronidase, and excessive occlusal forces. Bone re-

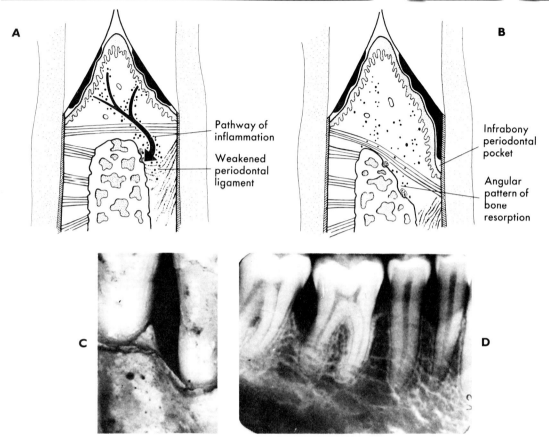

FIGURE 6-10. A, Inflammatory process may take the pathway in the interdental areas directly into the periodontal ligament when the crestal portion of the periodontal ligament has been weakened by excessive occlusal forces. **B,** Angular pattern of bone resorption and infrabony periodontal pockets are the result of the inflammatory process following the pathway directly into the periodontal ligament in the interdental areas. **C,** Angular pattern of bone resorption. **D,** Radiograph illustrating an angular pattern of bone loss on the distal aspects of the first premolar and the first molar.

sorption in periodontal disease is not a process of necrosis but one of viable cells destroying living bone.

Histopathology

The histological characteristics of periodontitis vary according to the length of time that the inflammatory process has been present; however, the typical characteristics of a mild to moder-

ately advanced periodontitis are as follows (Fig. 6-6, *B*):

1. Crevicular epithelium is ulcerated in some areas with deep spikes of epithelium proliferating into the connective tissue in other areas.
2. Junctional epithelium is located apical to the cementoenamel junction.
3. Immediately below the epithelium a

dense layer of chronic inflammation is noted by the following:

    a. Increase in the number of lymphocytes, plasma cells, and macrophages

    b. Dilation of blood vessels

    c. Disruption of gingival fibers (fibrinolysis)

4. Surrounding the zone of dense inflammation an area of mild cellular infiltration and pronounced proliferation of collagen fibers (fibrosis) is found.

5. Resorbing alveolar bone surfaces adjacent to the inflamed connective tissue and within the marrow spaces are characterized by osteoclasts (multinucleated cells) located in Howship's lacunae (shallow concave depressions in the bone) (Fig. 6-6, *B*).

Correlation of the histological findings with tissue changes noted clinically

During the early stages of gingival inflammation the tissue is red, soft, and boggy (edematous) because of the vascular stagnation, capillary proliferation, and breakdown of collagen fibers. However, as the disease becomes chronic, the inflammatory process tries to repair the destroyed tissue by stimulating fibroblasts to form more collagen fibers. This process masks the vascular changes, making the color of the tissue less red and the consistency more leathery (fibrotic). This stage persists until the disease becomes extremely advanced, when the edematous inflammatory changes may once again dominate the tissue response. An increase in the tendency to bleed from the gingival sulcus on gentle instrumentation is related to thinning of the crevicular epithelium, increased vascularity, and a close proximity of the engorged vessels to the pocket epithelium. The inner surface of the soft tissue pocket wall is somewhat painful to probing because of the ulceration of the crevicular epithelium. If purulent drainage is expressed from the pocket, it is related to suppurative inflammation of the inner wall of the pocket.

ETIOLOGY

The etiology of periodontitis is primarily related to the microorganisms and their products found in supra- and subgingival plaque. Common predisposing or secondary etiological factors that contribute to the accumulation, retention, and maturation of the plaque are supra- and subgingival deposits of calculus, overhanging gingival margins and overcontoured dental restorations leading to food impaction, and increased probing depths. Systemic factors may modify the body's tissue response to the bacteria. Therefore systemic factors can affect the severity of the periodontitis, but they do not initiate the inflammatory response.

Excessive occlusal forces can also play a modifying role in the progression of periodontitis by affecting the rate and pattern of tissue destruction. However, excessive occlusal forces have never been shown to initiate gingival inflammation or pocket formation. For a more detailed discussion of this subject refer to Chapter 2.

NUTRITIONAL IMPLICATIONS

Nutritional deficiencies can affect the way the gingival tissues react to the local irritating factors, but they have never been shown to cause gingival inflammation or to initiate or accelerate pocket formation in humans. For more details see Chapter 2. Since periodontitis is the result of a struggle between the pathological factors of the oral bacteria and the resistive and repair mechanisms of the host or periodontal tissues, an adequate dietary intake of the essential nutrients will have a favorable influence in preventing and recovering from periodontitis.

A soft, retentive diet, especially consisting of refined sugars, directly affects the development of gingivitis and periodontitis by enhancing bacterial growth and plaque formation.

PROGNOSIS

The outlook for retaining teeth in periodontal health that have been affected by periodontitis depends primarily on the ability of the patient and the dental team to control the etiological factors. It also depends on the amount of alveolar bone present, the number and distribution of the remaining teeth, and the magnitude of the occlusal demands placed on the dentition. If enough alveolar bone remains to support the teeth in function, the principal concerns are (1) whether the dentogingival environment is changed to reduce the retention of plaque (removal of calculus and other retentive factors and reduction in probing depths) and (2) whether the patient practices a level of plaque control consistent with periodontal health. If both occur the prognosis is generally favorable. However, if the etiological factors cannot be controlled because of inadequate patient cooperation with plaque control or uncontrollable systemic or occlusal factors, the prognosis is not favorable, and definitive periodontal treatment is not indicated.

The number and distribution of the remaining teeth are also important in determining the prognosis because occlusal forces and prosthetic abutments must be correctly distributed to prevent continued periodontal breakdown. For example, if the two mandibular cuspids and the two first molars are the only teeth that remain with adequate periodontal support, the prognosis for retaining them is favorable because occlusal forces can be distributed evenly on both sides of the dental arch. However, if the four teeth remaining are all in one posterior segment of one dental arch, the prognosis is poor because the mechanical forces of a prosthetic appliance cannot be distributed evenly over the entire dental arch, and the severe tipping forces of the appliance would contribute to continued periodontal tissue breakdown.

The magnitude of the occlusal forces placed on teeth can vary from patient to patient and affect the prognosis. If the patient has a habit of clenching or grinding the teeth, the bone support for the teeth will have to be greater than for a person who does not have these parafunctional habits. If the occlusal forces are excessive, the prognosis is often limited. (See Chapter 7.)

No specific heights of bone or depths of pockets always determine success or failure with periodontal treatment. Some teeth need more bone support than others to remain stable, and the depths of pockets do not necessarily represent the height of the periodontal attachment to the tooth. However, for a good prognosis, enough bone should remain to support the teeth in function, and the pockets must be able to be eliminated. If the pocket communicates with the apex of the tooth, the prognosis is usually not favorable, but endodontic therapy may improve the prognosis in some cases.

While the presence of purulent drainage (pus) in periodontal pockets indicates the presence of infection, it is not an indication of the amount of tissue destruction and therefore is not a definitive factor in prognosis.

A slight increase in tooth mobility (one degree) does not affect the prognosis significantly. However, a more severe increase (two degree mobility) usually makes the prognosis questionable, and if the tooth is depressible (three degree mobility), it is usually hopeless. The prognosis for reducing tooth mobility through periodontal therapy is related to the etiology of the mobility. Increased tooth movement may be related to inflammation in the gingiva and/or the periodontal ligament, the presence of occlusal trauma, loss of periodontal support (bone), or a combination of any of these factors. If the mobility is primarily related to inflammation, the prognosis for tightening the teeth through conventional periodontal therapy is fairly good. However, if the mobility is primarily related to occlusal trauma and/or loss of attachment, occlusal adjustment and/or splinting may be indicated as part of the therapy, and the long-range results are less predictable.

The one most important factor in achieving successful periodontal treatment is establishing good patient cooperation with plaque control. Without effective daily control of dental

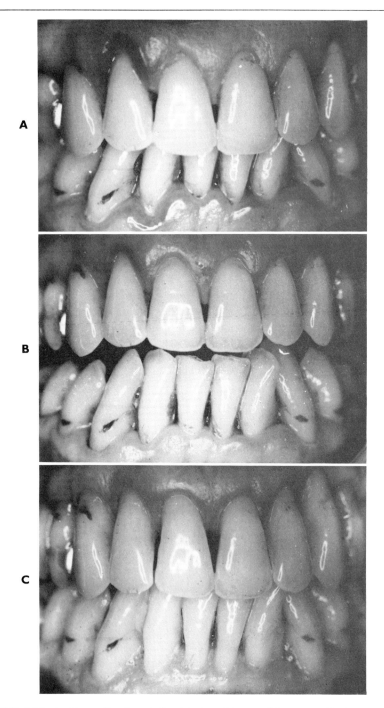

FIGURE 6-11. **A,** Generalized periodontitis in a 45-year-old woman. **B,** Same patient as in **A,** 1 month after instruction in oral hygiene and scaling and root planing of teeth. **C,** Same patient 1 year after periodontal surgery to correct the anatomical deformities (periodontal pockets and unfavorable gingival contours) created by the periodontitis.

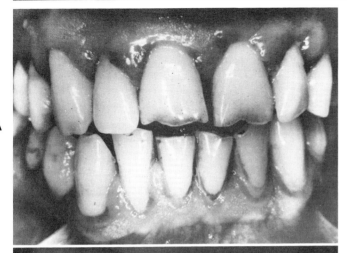

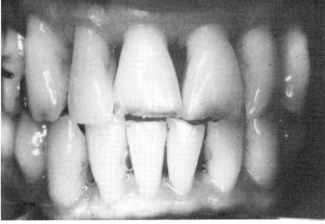

FIGURE 6-12. A, Moderate periodontitis in a 40-year-old man. Note soft bulbous contours of gingiva. **B,** Same patient as in **A** 3 years after periodontal surgery. Note the physiological contours of the gingiva.

plaque, the long-range prognosis is usually poor regardless of how severe the condition is when treatment is begun.

TREATMENT (Figs. 6-11 and 6-12)

Currently the treatment of periodontitis is principally aimed at reducing the amounts or changing the compositions of supra- and subgingival dental plaque to be compatible with periodontal health. Systemic causes when identified are also treated, but local therapy is usually necessary to control the bacteria that initiate the inflammation. The overall goal of treatment is to eliminate or at least minimize the inflammatory process in the gingiva.

This in turn eliminates the source of the inflammation and resorption in the deeper periodontal tissues. The periodontitis lesion tries to heal and repair itself, but because of continued irritation, the healing process is not allowed to go to completion. Periodontal treatment is concerned with creating a dentogingival environment that allows healing to take place.

The treatment of periodontitis can be divided into three basic phases:

Phase I   Initial periodontal treatment
Phase II   Correction of anatomical deformities
Phase III Maintenance periodontal treatment

Phase I is concerned with establishing rapport with the patient and eliminating as many of the etiological factors as possible without doing periodontal surgery or definitive restorative and prosthetic treatment (inlays, crowns, partial dentures, and so on). Following are some procedures done during this phase:

1. Patient education and instructions in plaque control
2. Scaling and root planing of teeth
3. Treatment of carious and endodontic lesions
4. Removal and provisional replacement of dental restorations and prosthetic appliances contributing to the periodontal disease
5. Preliminary occlusal adjustment
6. Temporary splinting of teeth
7. Orthodontics
8. Diet analysis and evaluation
9. Reevaluation of the periodontal status following the initial therapy to determine whether further treatment will be necessary.

Phase II includes the correction of anatomical deformities such as periodontal pockets, missing teeth, and occlusal disharmonies that have developed as a result of previous oral disease and may predispose to perpetuation or recurrence of periodontal disease. The following treatment procedures might be done during this phase:

1. Surgical reduction of pocket depths by one or more of the following methods:
   a. Gingival curettage
   b. Gingivectomy
   c. Periodontal flap procedures
   d. Osseous recontouring
   e. Periodontal regeneration procedures
2. Occlusal adjustment
3. Definitive dental and prosthetic restorations to create ideal tooth contours, interproximal contact points, and occlusal harmony and to replace missing teeth where indicated

Phase III maintenance periodontal treatment includes those procedures done periodically to help prevent the recurrence of the periodontal disease. The following are suggested treatment procedures:

1. Update of patient's medical and dental history
2. Reevaluation of periodontal health every 2 to 6 months by noting the plaque score, evidence of gingival inflammation, probing depths, and tooth mobility
3. Bite-wing radiographs taken at least once a year and full-mouth radiographic surveys every 3 to 4 years unless evidence of recurrent disease requires a more frequent evaluation
4. Review and reinforcement of the instructions in plaque control as needed every 2 to 6 months
5. Scaling and polishing of teeth every 2 to 6 months, depending on the effectiveness of the patient's plaque control and on the tendency to form calculus
6. Application of topical fluoride for patients susceptible to root caries

Recent research indicates that the benefits of periodontal surgical procedures are directly related to the effectiveness of the professional periodontal maintenance care received by the patient.

PATIENT EDUCATION

The success of periodontal treatment is intimately related to the patients' understanding of the cause of the disease and their willingness to perform those oral hygiene procedures necessary to maintain periodontal health.

Patients can learn about the nature and causes of periodontal disease through the use of commercially prepared films and publications. However, simple individualized illustrations and pointing out areas of health and disease in each patient's own mouth are particularly effective.

The details of implementing an effective plaque control program are described in Chapter 12. It is important to remember that patients should demonstrate the willingness and the ability to adequately control their dental plaque before any periodontal surgery is performed.

Many audiovisual aids and clever commercial products are available to facilitate patient education. However, if the dental team members demonstrate a sincerity in their recommendations by practicing effective plaque control and maintaining excellent dental health themselves, the patients' acceptance is rewarding. In designing an approach to patient education, remember that it is difficult to directly motivate anyone to do anything. However, through providing an environment for self-motivation the chances for long-range success in modifying oral hygiene habits is higher. One way to set up this environment during initial therapy is to have patients reduce gingival bleeding through improvement in their plaque control methods before the therapist removes the calculus and other irritating factors. This emphasizes the patients' role in controlling the periodontal disease.

PREVENTIVE MEASURES

Prevention of periodontitis is basically the prevention of gingivitis from developing into periodontitis. All gingivitis does not develop into periodontitis, but all periodontitis does begin as gingivitis. Why some cases of gingivitis develop into periodontitis and others do not is only partially understood. Changes in the patients' resistance may play a role, but it is reasonable to assume that the amount, composition, and location of the microorganisms in dental plaque are factors in the pathogenesis. The preventive methods discussed in this section are based on the assumption that continued accumulation and successive changes in the composition of the supra- and subgingival dental plaque are related to the development of gingivitis into periodontitis.

The prevention of gingivitis was discussed in Chapter 4 and essentially consists of providing a dentogingival environment conducive to adequate plaque control. This entails instructions in plaque control and the removal of tooth deposits and overhanging gingival margins. The prevention of gingivitis from developing into periodontitis involves definitively treating gingivitis, which is considered to be reversible, and correcting conditions that may predispose the patient to recurrent gingivitis or periodontitis. The preventive plan involves the following as indicated:

1. Establishment and maintenance of adequate plaque control by the patient
2. Effective removal of supra- and subgingival plaque and calculus by a dental professional at intervals frequent enough to prevent appreciable accumulations. The required time of the interval varies from one patient to another, but 3 months has been shown to be effective in preventing appreciable attachment loss in patients suseptible to periodontal disease.
3. Regular dental examinations to include updating of the patient's medical and dental histories and clinical condition enables the detection of early signs of gingival disease and definitive treatment before periodontitis develops.
4. Placement of dental prosthetic restorations with contours compatible with gingival health (avoiding overhanging gingival margins, open interproximal contact points, bulky contours, and partial dentures that impinge on the gingiva)
5. Orthodontics when indicated to provide tooth positions that do the following:
   a. Foster good gingival and periodontal anatomy
   b. Facilitate easy plaque control
   c. Direct occlusal forces along the long axes of the teeth
6. Evaluation of diet in the following areas:
   a. Nutrient intake
   b. Consistency of diet
   c. Frequency and form of sugar intake

SUGGESTED READINGS

Baer PN, and Norris ML: Textbook of periodontics, Philadelphia, 1977, JB Lippincott Co, pp 56-60, 96-132.

Carranza F: Glickman's clinical periodontology, ed 5, Philadelphia, 1979, WB Saunders Co, pp 209-267, 319-351.

Page R, and Schroeder H: Pathogenesis of inflammatory periodontal disease, Lab Invest 33:235, 1976.

Rosling B, et al: The healing potential of the periodontal tissues following different techniques of periodontal surgery in plaque free dentitions, J Clin Periodontol 3:233, 1976.

Schluger S, Yuodelis R, and Page R: Periodontal disease, Philadelphia, 1977, Lea &Febiger, Chapters 2 and 8.

CHAPTER 7
Early Onset Periodontitis

In recent years there has been a growing interest in the study of periodontitis as it affects children, adolescents, and young adults. Periodontitis in young individuals may be characterized by the large accumulations of dental plaque and calculus and slowly progressing bone resorption found in adult periodontitis. However, at least three other forms of periodontitis that affect this age group are particularly aggressive in terms of rapid bone resorption. They are collectively called early onset periodontitis and include the following:

1. Prepubertal periodontitis
2. Juvenile periodontitis (periodontosis)
3. Rapidly progressive periodontitis

PREPUBERTAL PERIODONTITIS

Prepubertal periodontitis is an unusual disease that results in the resorption of the periodontal tissues in young children during or shortly following the eruption of the primary teeth. The disease leads to early loss of the deciduous teeth and may affect the permanent dentition as well. Based on clinical symptoms there are localized and generalized forms of the disease.

In the localized form there are minimal clinical signs of gingival inflammation and only some of the teeth are involved (Fig. 7-1). The rate of tissue destruction is slower than in the generalized form. The etiology of this condition is not fully known, but a defect in the patient's ability to resist the effect of the plaque microorganisms is suspected. In the localized form, the leukocyte (white blood cell) defects involve the polymorphonuclear leukocytes or mononu-

clear leukocytes, but not both. Polymorphonuclear leukocytes are considered to be an important first line of defense in the gingiva. Abnormal cementum formation or maintenance which creates a defective periodontal attachment may lower the resistance of the periodontal tissues to microbial infection and allow rapid tissue destruction. This form of the disease responds well to local mechanical debridement of the affected sites combined with the systemic administration of antibiotics. The drugs of choice are penicillin or erythromycin administered in doses of 250 mg four times a day for 3 weeks.

Generalized prepubertal periodontitis is characterized clinically by severe inflammation and bone resorption around all the primary teeth and leads to their early exfoliation. The permanent dentition may also be affected, but because of the small number of cases reported information is limited on the long-range effects of the disease. Patients with this condition generally exhibit defects in both the polymorphonuclear and the mononuclear leukocytes. This disease is often associated with frequent abscess formation, upper respiratory tract infections, and otitis media. Local treatment is not enhanced by the administration of antibiotics.

The American Academy of Periodontology suggests in a 1987 position paper that patients with affected primary dentitions who have systemic diseases such as neutropenia, agranulocytosis, aplastic anemia, hypophosphatasia, or Papillon-Lefévre syndrome should be differentiated from patients with prepubertal periodontitis.

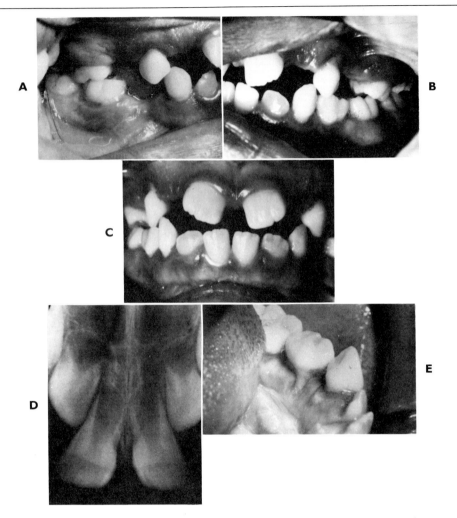

FIGURE 7-1. A-H, Prepubertal periodontitis in 6-year-old girl. (Courtesy Dr. Keiko Watanabe)

JUVENILE PERIODONTITIS (PERIODONTOSIS)
Definition

Juvenile periodontitis refers to an uncommon form of periodontitis seen in children and adolescents. It is characterized by rapid alveolar bone destruction with minimal signs of gingival inflammation. It is classified into localized and generalized forms based on its distribution in the dentition. The incidence of the disease is less than 1% in developed nations and in the range of 5% in underdeveloped regions.

Periodontosis was a term used to describe a form of periodontal disease that results in the rapid loss of the periodontal tissues around more than one permanent tooth in otherwise healthy adolescents and young adults. The suffix -osis was used in the name of this condition because in the early stages of the disease the primary pathological tissue changes were con-

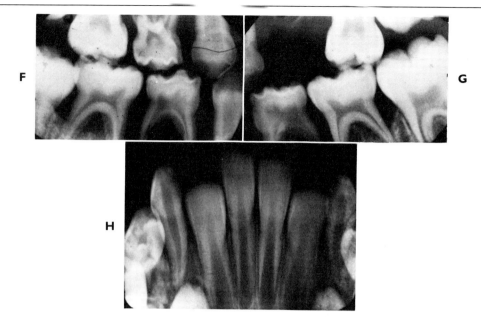

FIGURE 7-1, cont'd. For legend see opposite page.

sidered to be degenerative rather than inflammatory *(-itis)*. Scientific investigations have not substantiated the early degenerative changes in this condition and this term is no longer considered appropriate. Current evidence suggests that the condition classically described as periodontosis is more correctly termed the localized form of juvenile periodontitis.

Clinical characteristics
Generalized form

The generalized form affects the entire dentition and is frequently associated with systemic conditions such as hypophosphatasia, Down's syndrome, and Papillon-Lefévre syndrome. It can, however, occur in an individual with no apparent systemic disease and is characterized by advanced periodontal tissue loss, pathological tooth migration, increased tooth mobility, severe gingival inflammation, and periodontal pocket formation.

Papillon-Lefévre syndrome is characterized by hyperkeratotic scaly skin lesions combined with severe periodontal destruction, frequently beginning before the age of 4 years. The skin lesions are typically found on the palms of the hands and soles of the feet. The periodontal lesions involve early inflammatory tissue changes, leading to the exfoliation of the primary teeth by 5 or 6 years of age and the loss of the permanent dentition by age 15.

Hypophosphatasia is a rare familial skeletal condition that may result in the loss of the primary dentition.

Down's syndrome (mongolism) is a congenital disease caused by a chromosomal abnormality and involves mental deficiency and growth retardation. The periodontal disease seen in these patients is caused primarily by plaque and calculus, but the tissue destruction frequently exceeds what can be related to local irritating factors alone.

Localized form

The localized form of juvenile periodontitis is more closely related to the classic description

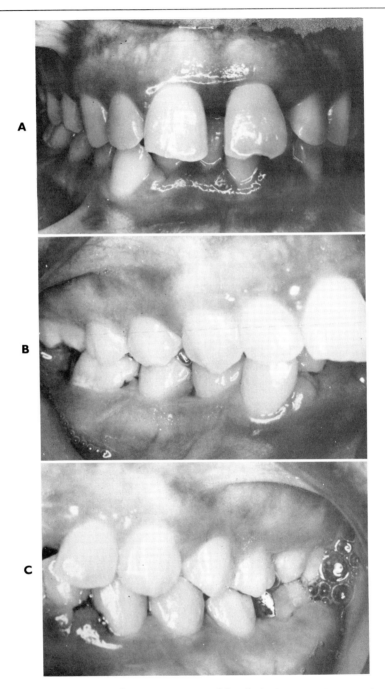

FIGURE 7-2. Juvenile periodontitis in 16-year-old girl. **A,** Anterior view showing pathological migration of central incisiors. **B,** Right side of dentition; note minimal signs of gingival inflammation on posterior teeth. **C,** Left side of dentition; note minimal signs of gingival inflammation on posterior teeth.

of periodontosis. It is characterized by rapid alveolar bone destruction and deep infrabony pocket formation on the permanent incisors and first molars from puberty to 25 years of age. During the early phases the disease is frequently not recognized because the gingiva appears to be healthy. Labial migration of the maxillary incisors is also a frequent finding (Fig. 7-2). While minimal amounts of plaque and calculus are seen during the early phases of the disease, if the pockets have been present for several years, plaque, calculus, and gingival inflammation will be more evident.

While both males and females are affected by this disease, the incidence is higher in females. Members of the same family are frequently affected. The deciduous dentition is not affected.

Radiographic signs
Generalized form

Advanced alveolar bone loss occurs around all or most of the teeth. Both the primary and the permanent dentition may be affected.

Localized form

Angular or vertical alveolar bone loss occurs around the permanent first molars and incisors (Figs. 7-3 and 7-4). An arc-shaped pattern of bone loss extends from the distal aspect of the second premolar to the mesial aspect of the second molar. Bilateral bone loss is common.

Histopathology and pathogenesis

While the exact pathogenesis of juvenile periodontitis is not confirmed, current concepts suggest that the disease begins in the gingival tissues and migrates apically to destroy the bone and periodontal ligament and form deep infrabony pockets. No explanation yet exists as to why the incisors and first molars are primarily affected.

Etiology

Definitive etiological factors are not known at this time, but the predominant thinking is that the principal cause is bacterial with the possibility of an altered host response. The following factors are implicated:

1. Unusual bacterial flora are found in the periodontal pockets with an increased

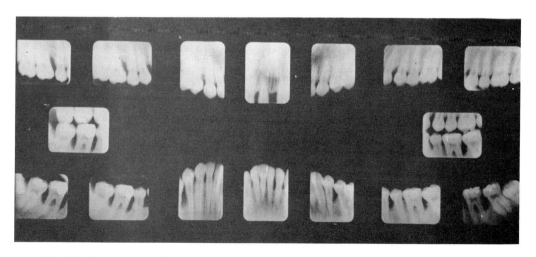

FIGURE 7-3. Radiographs of patient in Fig. 7-2. Note advanced angular bone loss on the incisor and first molar teeth.

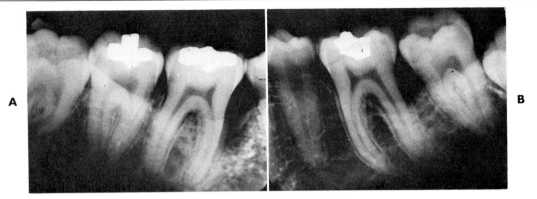

FIGURE 7-4. Angular bone loss patterns in 17-year-old boy. **A,** Mandibular right first molar. **B,** Mandibular left first molar.

proportion of gram-negative anaerobic rods. (Organisms of healthy gingival sulci are predominantly gram-positive.)

2. The presence of two microorganisms that are capable of causing rapid destruction of the periodontal tissues are prominently increased. *Actinobacillus actinomycetemcomitans* is a leukotoxin producer, and *Capnocytophaga sputigena* produces an antineutrophil factor.

3. Impaired neutrophil chemotaxis lowers the patient's resistance to bacterial infection and allows more rapid tissue destruction.

4. More intense immune response than that found in periodontitis is seen, therefore resulting in more severe destruction of the periodontal tissues.

5. Familial involvement is reported, with the condition occurring in identical twins, parents and offspring, siblings, first cousins, uncles and nephews.

Nutritional implications

No nutritional deficiencies have been established in relation to juvenile periodontitis.

Prognosis

The prognosis for long-term maintenance of health in teeth and periodontal tissues affected by juvenile periodontitis varies from questionable to hopeless, depending on the extent of the bone destruction and the etiological factors involved. The uncertainty of the causative factors makes treatment less than definitive and of limited effectiveness. However, if the disease is treated early enough with plaque control and pocket elimination, the teeth can sometimes be preserved for many years. In certain cases the incisors and first molars have a poor prognosis, but the remainder of the dentition has a good prognosis. Some patients also show a decrease in the rate of bone loss in their middle and late twenties. Because of the individual variation in cases, it is important to determine the prognosis for each case individually.

Treatment

In view of the fact that the etiology of juvenile periodontitis is still speculative, the treatment procedures are basically empirical. Several different approaches have been developed and include the following:

1. Selective extraction and replacement of the severely involved teeth. This is applicable when the disease is localized to the first molars and incisors.

2. Scaling and root planing of the teeth and surgical curettement of the periodontal pocket with the intent of stimulating the

regeneration of lost periodontal attachment tissues. Systemic administration of the antibiotic tetracycline appears to be a useful adjunct to the local instrumentation therapy. The periodontopathic organisms in localized juvenile periodontitis are particularly sensitive to tetracycline. Suggested dosage of tetracycline is 250 mg, 1 tablet every 6 hours for 3 weeks.

3. Surgical curettement of the periodontal pocket combined with reshaping the occlusal surface of the involved teeth to temporarily remove all occlusal contacts. This allows eruption of the involved tooth. As the tooth erupts, the alveolar bone directly attached to the periodontal ligament is stimulated to move coronally with the tooth and thereby help to make the infrabony defects more shallow. The occlusal adjustment is done several times at weekly intervals to stimulate continued eruption of the tooth.

4. Conventional surgical pocket elimination including periodontal flap procedures, osseous recontouring, and root amputations where needed. This method of treatment is indicated in the patients with generalized pocketing and bone loss and in situations in which the osseous recontouring will not seriously jeopardize the supporting tissues of the adjacent teeth.

5. Selective extraction and replacement of seriously involved molar teeth by autotransplantation of developing third molars. These procedures have also been done for patients with advanced lesions around the first molars.

6. Periodic scaling, curettage, and meticulous oral hygiene. The rationale for this method of treatment is that the rapid destruction of tissue associated with this disease may be diminished as the patient matures, and definitive pocket elimination may be more effectively performed at that time.

7. Extraction of all teeth and replacement with complete dentures. This procedure is indicated for patients with generalized advanced bone loss and for those who do not respond to conventional periodontal treatment.

8. Two-stage approach for patients who require prophylactic antibiotic therapy to prevent endocarditis. Tetracycline hydrochloride therapy (1 g/day) for 14 days before periodontal treatment is used to suppress the *Actinobacillus actinomycetemcomitans,* and then the conventional prophylactic protocol (penicillin or erythromycin) is followed to reduce the streptococci during the time of dental treatment.

While definitive treatment of patients with juvenile periodontitis is sometimes discouraging, the success ratio is high enough to warrant periodontal treatment in many patients, and routine extraction of all teeth involved with this condition cannot be justified.

Patient education

Patients should be informed of the nature and prognosis of the disease and of their role in helping to control the local irritants. Specific instructions do not differ from those given to a patient being treated for advanced periodontitis.

Preventive measures

No definitive preventive procedures for juvenile periodontitis exist because the etiological factors are not known. However, periodontal treatment of the early lesions helps prevent the continued progression of periodontal tissue destruction in some patients.

RAPIDLY PROGRESSIVE PERIODONTITIS

Rapidly progressive periodontitis, most frequently seen in patients in their twenties, is a condition in which there is extensive bone resorption in a short period of time. The disease may begin any time between puberty and 30 to

35 years of age. This disease may be related to the generalized form of juvenile periodontitis. The disease progression is episodic with periods of exacerbation followed by remission. The clinical characteristics of the acute phases of the disease include highly inflamed gingiva that bleeds easily and has a mulberry-like surface. The amount of plaque present is variable. The quiescent phase is characterized by normal gingival appearances and tissues that are tightly attached to the teeth even though advanced bone loss and deep periodontal pockets persist. This dormant phase may be permanent or temporary. The active phase may also be accompanied by malaise, weight loss, and depression.

Most patients with these conditions manifest defects in either neutrophil or monocyte chemotaxis and their compromised defense systems may partly account for the symptoms noted. The bacterial flora associated with this disease have not been definitively identified, but the following are implicated as important pathogens: gram-negative, anaerobic, asaccharolytic rods, especially *Bacteroides*, *Actinobacillus*, and possibly *Capnocytophaga*.

Several systemic diseases are known to be associated with rapid periodontal tissue destruction and may predispose or be related to rapidly progressive periodontitis. Examples are diabetes mellitus, Down's syndrome, Crohn's disease, neutropenia, agranulocytosis, the lazy leukocyte syndrome, and the Chediak-Higashi syndrome.

Most patients with rapidly progressive periodontitis not associated with a known systemic disease respond favorably to treatment by scaling and open or closed curettage when accompanied by antibiotic therapy. However, a small number of patients do not respond to any forms of periodontal therapy, and the teeth are lost. Unfortunately it is not possible to distinguish prior to treatment which patients will respond to therapy and which will not.

SUGGESTED READINGS

Baer PN, and Morris M: Textbook of periodontics, Philadelphia, 1977, JB Lippincott Co, pp 323-330.

Carranza F: Glickman's clinical periodontology, ed 5, Philadelphia, 1979, WB Saunders Co, pp 201-207, 309-316.

Genco R: Antibiotics in the treatment of human periodontal diseases, J Periodontol 52:545, 1981.

Newman M, and Socransky S: Predominant cultivable microbiota in periodontosis, J Periodont Res 12:120, 1977.

Page RC, and Baab DA: A new look at the etiology and pathogenesis of early onset periodontitis. Cementopathia revisited, J Periodontol 56:748-751, 1985.

Page RC, et al: Prepubertal periodontitis. I. Definition of a clinical entity, J Periodontol 54:257-271, 1983.

Page RC, et al: Rapidly progressive periodontitis: A distinct clinical condition J Periodontol 54:197-209, 1983.

Schluger S, Yuodelis R, and Page R: Periodontal disease, Philadelphia, 1977, Lea & Febiger, pp 69-71.

Slots J, Rosling B, and Genco R: Suppression of penicillin-resistant oral *Actinobacillus actinomycetemcomitans* with tetracycline considerations in endocarditis prophylaxis, J Periodontol 54:193, 1983.

Slots J, et al: *Actinobacillus actinomycetemcomitans* in human periodontal disease, J Periodont Res 17:447, 1982.

CHAPTER 8
Periodontal Occlusal Trauma

DEFINITION

Periodontal occlusal trauma is the degenerative lesion that develops when occlusal forces exceed the adaptive capacity of the supporting periodontal tissues. It is characterized by breakdown of the periodontal ligament fibers, bone resorption, widening of the periodontal ligament space, and loosening of the teeth.

Occlusal trauma in the periodontal tissues has been classified as primary and secondary. *Primary occlusal trauma* results when increases in the magnitude and/or the duration of occlusal forces or change in the direction of the forces become excessive in the presence of normal periodontal tissue support (Fig. 8-1). *Secondary occlusal trauma* develops when the normal forces of occlusion become excessive because of severe loss of periodontal support rather than an increase in the occlusal forces (Fig. 8-2).

This chapter is devoted only to the periodontal tissue changes that occur when occlusal forces become excessive. Occlusal wearing of the teeth, pulpal changes, and muscle spasms as well as pain in the temporomandibular joint can also occur as the result of occlusal disharmonies. While these topics are not discussed in this book, it should be remembered that periodontal occlusal trrauma may be only one of the clinical manifestations of occlusal trauma.

CLINICAL CHARACTERISTICS

The clinical characteristics of periodontal occlusal trauma vary according to the severity of the excessive forces and the length of time the changes have been present. The symptoms be-

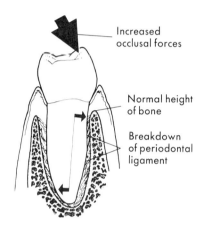

FIGURE 8-1. Primary occlusal trauma. Breakdown of the periodontal ligament is related to an increase in the magnitude and/or duration of occlusal forces, or a change in the direction of the forces.

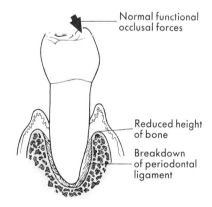

FIGURE 8-2. Secondary occlusal trauma. Breakdown of the periodontal ligament occurs as a result of the normal functional forces of occlusion becoming excessive because of the advanced loss of bone support.

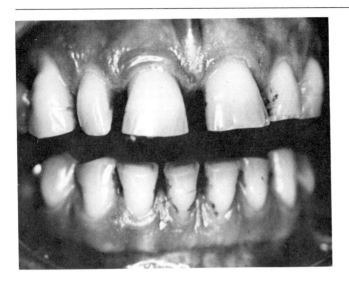

FIGURE 8-3. Flaring of the anterior teeth related to loss of posterior tooth support, parafunctional habits, and resultant occlusal trauma. No periodontal pockets are present in this 42-year-old woman.

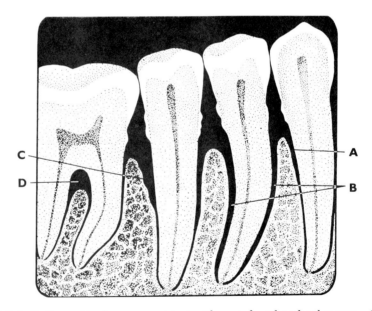

FIGURE 8-4. Radiographic changes consistent with periodontal occlusal trauma. **A,** Widening of the crestal portion of the periodontal ligament space. **B,** Irregular widening of the entire periodontal ligament space. Radiographic changes consistent with periodontal occlusal trauma combined with periodontitis: **C,** Angular pattern of bone loss. **D,** Radiolucency in the furcations.

low, however, are commonly associated with both primary and secondary occlusal trauma:

1. Increasing mobility of the teeth
2. Fremitus (a palpable or visible movement of a tooth when subjected to occlusal forces)
3. Migration of teeth (Fig. 8-3)
4. Sensitivity of the teeth to pressure

RADIOGRAPHIC CHANGES (Figs. 8-4 and 8-5)

The following radiographic changes may be found:

1. Widening of the crestal portion of the periodontal ligament space (Figs. 8-4, A, and 8-5, A)
2. Irregular widening of the entire periodontal ligament space (Figs. 8-4, B, and 8-5, B)
3. If periodontitis is also present, there is a tendency for a vertical or angular pattern of bone loss and radiolucencies in the furcation areas (Figs. 8-4, C and D, 8-5, C and D)

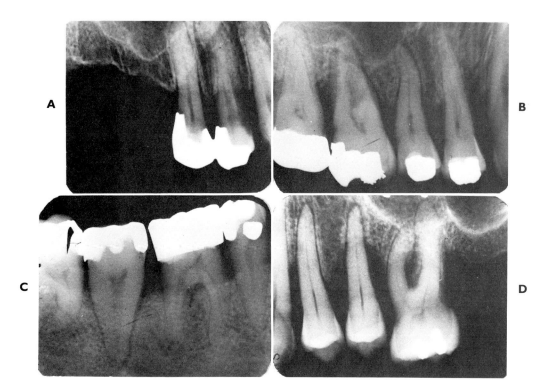

FIGURE 8-5. Radiographic changes associated with periodontal occlusal trauma alone. **A,** Widening of the crestal portion of the periodontal ligament space. **B,** Irregular widening of the entire periodontal ligament space (note second premolar and first molar). **C,** Irregular widening of the periodontal ligament space on a second molar and radiolucency in the furcation area of the first molar. **D,** Angular pattern of bone loss on the second premolar and a radiolucency in the furcation of the first molar consistent with occlusal trauma combined with periodontitis.

HISTOPATHOLOGY AND PATHOGENESIS

Occlusal functional stimulation is essential for the maintenance of a well-structured, healthy periodontal ligament and alveolar bone. The lack of occlusal forces results in *periodontal atrophy* characterized by loosely arranged periodontal ligament fibers, decreased density of the bone trabeculation patterns, and thinning of the periodontal ligament spaces. These changes are seen in teeth that have lost their opponents. Clinically periodontal atrophy becomes important when the tooth is placed back in function as a bridge abutment or as an opponent for a prosthetic appliance. The tooth may be painful and slightly mobile until the periodontal tissues are reorganized into a well-structured functioning unit.

In contrast to the need for occlusal stimulation to maintain periodontal health, in certain circumstances occlusal forces can be damaging to the periodontium and cause the development of periodontal occlusal trauma. This condition can result from an increase or a change in the direction of the forces placed on teeth (primary) or from the loss of supporting tissues (secondary), making the normal forces of occlusion too much for the remaining periodontium to withstand. In either case the tissue changes in the periodontal ligament are similar in that they go through degenerative and adaptive phases. During the degenerative phase the periodontal ligament fibers are crushed and torn, the blood vessels become thrombosed, the alveolar bone undergoes osteoclastic resorption making the periodontal ligament space wider, and the cementum is sometimes torn. An influx of inflammatory cells in the periodontal ligament space is absent, and no gingival or junctional epithelium changes have ever been seen histologically that can be related to excessive occlusal forces. However, the periodontal tissues have the capacity to adjust to excessive occlusal forces. This is called the *adaptive phase* and is characterized by a widening of the periodontal ligament space, longer periodontal ligament fibers, normal vasculature, and a normal alveolar bone proper. The tooth may have an increase in mobility and may have shifted in position to avoid the excessive occlusal forces, but active occlusal trauma will not be present. This phenomenon illustrates the capacity of the periodontium to heal and adjust to the increased occlusal forces. Occlusal trauma, therefore, does not have to be a progressively destructive lesion. In addition, if the occlusal forces can be altered or the periodontal tissue resistance can be increased to bring the occlusal forces back into the range of the adaptive capacity of the periodontium, the tissue changes of occlusal trauma are reversible.

The gingiva and junctional epithelium are not directly affected in this lesion because the only way excessive occlusal forces can cause damage is by crushing or tearing tissues located in or adjacent to a confined area, namely the periodontal ligament space. The gingiva is not susceptible to these forces, and this is why pocket formation cannot be initiated by excessive occlusal forces. However, when inflammatory changes are also present in the periodontium as a result of local irritation, the occlusal trauma can lower the resistance of the deep periodontal tissues to pocket formation, and a tendency for more rapid tissue destruction is seen. The pockets may be of the infrabony type because under these circumstances it is postulated that the inflammatory process tends to spread directly into the periodontal ligament, causing resorption of the alveolar bone proper before the more superficial supporting bone. (See Figs. 6-9 and 6-10.) While tissue changes associated with occlusal trauma alone are reversible, those related to both occlusal trauma and inflammation are not.

ETIOLOGY

The etiological factors of periodontal occlusal trauma can be divided into four categories:

1. Situations that increase the magnitude or frequency of occlusal forces
2. Situations that change the direction of occlusal forces
3. Circumstances that reduce the resistance of the periodontium to occlusal forces
4. Combinations of any of these factors

Situations that increase the magnitude or frequency of occlusal forces

1. Long-sustained and increased magnitude of occlusal contacts during parafunctional habits such as clenching, bruxism, and chewing on pipe stem*
2. Restorative and prosthetic dentistry that does not harmonize with the entire occlusion and directs the entire occlusal load onto one or a few teeth
3. Fixed and removable prosthetic appliances

Situations that change the direction of occlusal forces so that they are not directed along the long axes of the teeth

1. Tipping forces from occlusal interferences such as centric prematurities and balancing side contacts, which usually occur on inclined planes
2. Parafunctional habits in extreme eccentric positions
3. Poorly designed restorative and prosthetic treatments that generate tipping occlusal forces
4. Tilting and drifting of teeth

Circumstances that reduce the resistance of the periodontium to occlusal forces

1. Loss of alveolar bone and periodontal ligament support

---

*Because of reflex mechanisms the occlusal forces generated during mastication, swallowing, and talking are usually short in duration and light in pressure. They are therefore of little significance in the generation of an increase in the magnitude of occlusal forces.

2. Loss of a number of teeth, thereby requiring fewer teeth to absorb the entire occlusal load

An increase in the magnitude and a change in the direction of the occlusal forces as well as a reduction in periodontal resistance are commonly found in patients who have moderate to advanced periodontitis combined with missing and drifted teeth, occlusal disharmonies, and parafunctional habits.

While the preceding factors have the potential to cause occlusal trauma, because of the range of adaptation of the periodontal tissues, these situations do not always result in degenerative periodontal tissue changes. For example, it has been shown that a large number of young adults have centric prematurities, but only a small number of this age group have clinical evidence of periodontal occlusal trauma. In addition, some patients who have a habit of bruxism cause severe wearing away of the teeth rather than periodontal occlusal trauma.

NUTRITIONAL IMPLICATIONS

Severe deficiencies in protein, calcium, and vitamin D may exaggerate the severity of a periodontal occlusal trauma lesion, but nutritional deficiencies have not been shown to cause occlusal trauma.

PROGNOSIS

The outlook for retaining teeth that are affected in periodontal occlusal trauma depends on the degree of control the dentist has over the etiological factors and the severity of the periodontal tissue loss.

If the occlusal trauma is related to a restoration that was placed in supraocclusion, the prognosis is favorable because the dentist has control over the occlusal contours of restorations. Also, if the occlusal trauma is related to reduced periodontal support, splinting and replacement of missing teeth can often control the occlusal trauma for long periods. However, if the occlusal trauma is caused primarily by parafunctional habits related to nervous tension, the outlook for reducing the increased occlusal forces is not favorable. The prognosis for successfully treating occlusal trauma frequently depends on the restorative and prosthetic portions of the treatment, which are beyond the scope of this book.

TREATMENT

The treatment for periodontal occlusal trauma depends on the etiology as well as the type of lesion and how advanced it is.

Primary occlusal trauma is usually treated by one or more of the following procedures:

1. Occlusal adjustment by reshaping to eliminate occlusal discrepancies
2. Orthodontic tooth movement to realign the occlusal forces in a more axial direction
3. Bite planes, night guards, and/or stress reduction programs when necessary to eliminate or reduce parafunctional habits
4. Occlusal rehabilitation to eliminate occlusal discrepancies and to realign the direction of occlusal forces

These procedures may also be used in the management of secondary occlusal trauma. However, the principal concern in the treatment of secondary occlusal trauma is increasing the resistance of the periodontal supporting tissues to occlusal forces. Splinting teeth, which is often used in the treatment of secondary occlusal trauma, has the effect of increasing the number of roots per tooth and changing the center of tooth rotation so that occlusal forces are more favorably received and dissipated. The splints may be temporary or permanent, fixed or removable.

The treatment of occlusal trauma should only be done with an awareness of the manifestations on the entire stomatognathic system. A detailed discussion on this subject is beyond the scope of this book.

PATIENT EDUCATION

The patient should be informed about the nature of occlusal trauma and the rationale for the treatment. If removable appliances such as bite plates and night guards are used in the treatment, definite instructions on their use and care should be given to the patient.

PREVENTIVE MEASURES

The prevention of periodontal occlusal trauma involves eliminating the etiological factors before they cause the lesion. This may involve some or all of the following procedures:

1. As many teeth as possible should be preserved and those teeth that are lost should be replaced if they are needed to maintain the integrity of the arch.
2. Periodontal disease should be treated early to prevent extreme bone loss and loss of teeth.
3. Restorative and prosthetic appliances should be placed in such a way that they do not create occlusal discrepancies or cause severe nonaxial loading.
4. Orthodontics should be performed to assure that occlusal forces are directed as much as possible on the long axes of the teeth and to eliminate occlusal discrepancies.
5. Occlusal adjustment by reshaping to eliminate centric prematurities and interferences in the excursive movements is occasionally indicated on a preventive basis, for example, following orthodontics or before extensive restorative dentistry. However, in general, if no evidence of pathology related to the occlusal discrepancies exists, occlusal adjustment should *not* be done with the hope that it will prevent occlusal trauma in the future. Research evidence has not shown that occlusal discrepancies such as centric prematurities predictably cause occlusal trauma. In addition, the possibility of

creating a "positive occlusal sense" after the occlusal adjustment is another contraindication. A "positive occlusal sense" refers to the situation when people are always aware of their occlusion. It is particularly unfortunate when this happens in a patient who had no symptoms before the occlusal adjustment.

SUGGESTED READINGS

Carranza F: Glickman's clinical periodontology, ed 5, Philadelphia, 1979, WB Saunders Co, pp 275-293.

Ramfjord S, and Ash M: Occlusion, ed 2, Philadelphia, 1971, WB Saunders Co, pp 158-174.

Zander H, and Polson A: Present status of occlusion and occlusal therapy in periodontics, J Periodontol 48:540, 1977.

CHAPTER 9
Gingival Recession

DEFINITIONS

Gingival recession refers to a progressive exposure of the tooth's root surface resulting from apical migration of the junctional epithelium and gingiva. This term denotes a comparable resorption of alveolar bone and periodontal ligament as well (Fig. 9-1).

Stillman's clefts are a specific type of gingival recession characterized by narrow slits that run in an apical direction from the marginal gingiva (Fig. 9-2).

CLINICAL CHARACTERISTICS (Fig. 9-3)

Gingival recession is noted clinically by having the crest of the marginal gingiva located apical to the cementoenamel junction. The tissues may be red and inflamed or pink and firm, depending on the amount of local irritants present. In either situation the gingiva is usually thin and friable with little or no attached gingiva. While pocket formation may accompany this condition, the depth of the gingival sulcus is often within normal limits.

The teeth are often prominently positioned in the arch as they relate to the adjacent teeth. Gingival recession can occur at any age, but it occurs more frequently with increased age.

RADIOGRAPHIC FINDINGS

No radiographic findings are characteristic of gingival recession on the facial and lingual surfaces of teeth. Soft tissue changes and the facial and lingual plates of alveolar bone are not usually depicted on a dental radiograph. Generalized periodontal recession including the loss of interproximal supporting structures as well as

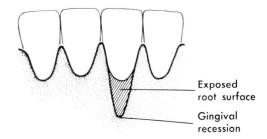

FIGURE 9-1. Gingival recession on the facial surface of a mandibular central incisor. Note the exposed root surface.

the facial and lingual tissues can be recognized on the radiograph by reduction of the height of the alveolar process in relationship to the cementoenamel junction.

HISTOPATHOLOGY AND PATHOGENESIS

The mechanism whereby gingival recession occurs is not completely understood. A certain amount of gingival recession may be part of aging and the normal result of passive eruption. However, some researchers consider any recession a pathological change. In either case the process consists of progressive apical migration of the junctional epithelium and an accompanying destruction of the gingiva, alveolar bone, and periodontal ligament.

Gingival recession is often the result of the inflammatory tissue changes associated with periodontitis. However, gingival recession also occurs when the tissues appear to be healthy. Toothbrush trauma and an accompanying destruction of the periodontium may take place

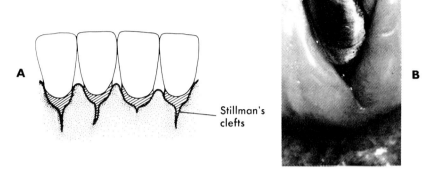

FIGURE 9-2. A, Stillman's clefts. This type of gingival recession is characterized by narrow slits that run in an apical direction from the marginal gingiva. **B,** Stillman's clefts in 47-year-old man.

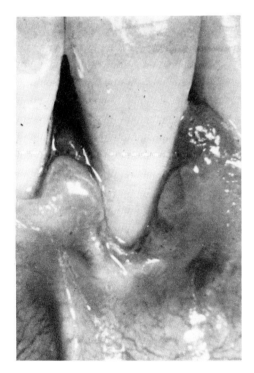

FIGURE 9-3. Isolated gingival recession on tooth 24. Note the rounded edematous tissue and the lack of attached gingiva. The patient is 18 years old.

even though the tissues appear clinically to remain uninflamed (Fig. 9-4).

ETIOLOGY

While the exact etiology of gingival recession is not known, following are some of the factors considered important in the development of this condition:

1. Bacterial plaque can cause inflammatory tissue changes and destruction (Fig. 9-5).
2. Uneven gingival margins (Fig. 9-6), over-contoured restorations, and overhanging gingival margins can accentuate the localized accumulation of dental plaque and thereby contribute to the etiology of localized periodontal inflammation and recession.
3. Prosthetic appliances can impinge on the gingiva (Fig. 9-7).
4. Toothbrushing can cause abrasion, especially using a hard toothbrush and a horizontal scrubbing motion (Fig. 9-4).
5. Prominent tooth positioning in the dental arch predisposes to recession by creating thin periodontal tissues and alveolar bone dehiscences (Figs. 9-8 and 9-9).

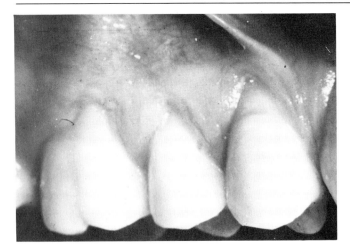

FIGURE 9-4. Cervical abrasion of the teeth and accompanying gingival recession in a 16-year-old boy.

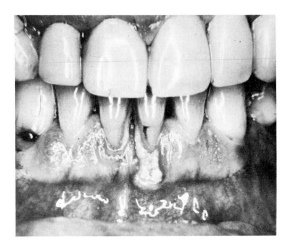

FIGURE 9-5. Isolated area of gingival recession related primarily to the accumulation of bacterial plaque and associated oral debris.

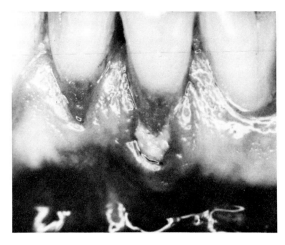

FIGURE 9-6. Uneven gingival margins contributing to plaque accumulation.

6. Excessive occlusal forces may cause resorption of thin facial or lingual radicular bone and thereby predispose the overlying gingiva to recession. However, excessive occlusal forces do not directly cause apical migration of the junctional epithelium and gingival recession.
7. Frena or muscle attachments can undermine the marginal tissues and change the connective tissue composition from the dense collagen mass found in gingiva to loosely arranged muscle and elastic fibers characteristic of alveolar mucosa. The resultant thin, loosely attached tissue creates a sulcus that seems to accumulate plaque easily and cause inflammation (Figs. 9-10 and 9-11).
8. Inadequate zones of attached gingiva

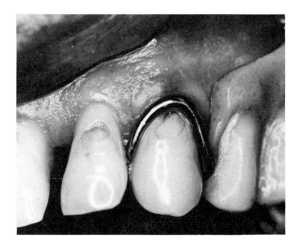

FIGURE 9-7. Partial denture clasp placed too close to the gingival margin.

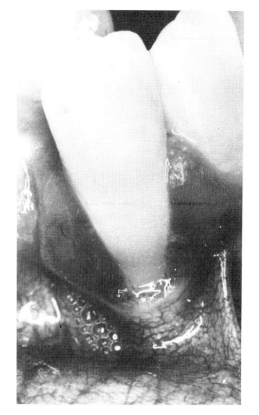

FIGURE 9-8. Note the labial tilting of tooth 25 with the resulting thin tissue covering on the facial surface. No attached gingiva is present in this area.

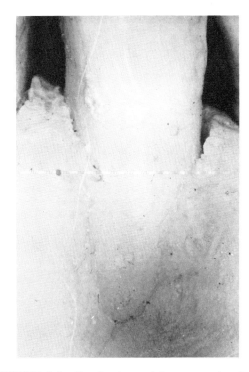

FIGURE 9-9. Alveolar bone dehiscence related to the prominent position of the tooth in the dental arch. This can be a predisposing factor in the etiology of gingival recession.

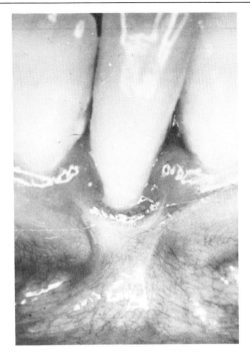

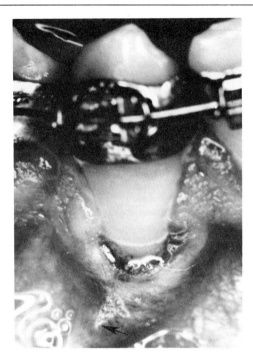

FIGURE 9-10. Attachment of the mandibular labial frenum into the marginal gingiva of tooth 25. This eliminates the attached gingiva and predisposes the area to gingival recession.

FIGURE 9-11. Note the insertion of the muscle fiber into the marginal gingiva on the facial of tooth 27 (arrow).

cause oral mucosa to serve as the marginal tissue around a tooth. Compared to attached gingiva, this loosely attached, nonkeratinized tissue is not as well-suited to act as marginal tissue. This is because it does not withstand well the forces of toothbrushing and food skirting over it during mastication. While inadequate zones of attached gingiva may predispose the area to gingival recession, research indicates that if effective plaque control is practiced in these areas, attachment levels can be maintained.

9. Gingiva that is habitually injured with fingernails, pencils, hairpins, and other sharp objects may cause recession.

NUTRITIONAL IMPLICATIONS

No nutritional factors associated with gingival recession are known.

PROGNOSIS

The outlook for preventing further loss of tissue in areas of gingival recession depends primarily on maintaining the tissues free of inflammation along with the severity and etiology of the recession.

In general, if the recession is not too extensive and the etiological factors can be identified and corrected, the prognosis for preventing further recession is favorable.

Of particular concern is the maintenance of a level of nontraumatic plaque control that is consistent with gingival health and, where necessary, the reestablishment of an adequate zone of attached gingiva and a tooth position and contour located within the alveolar housing.

The restoration of gingiva on root surfaces previously denuded by recession is possible and is indicated when gingival health cannot be established because of a mucogingival defect or for esthetic reasons. If an adequate zone of attached gingiva is present on an adjacent tooth, a pedicle flap can be positioned over the exposed root, and the outlook for covering it is quite good (see Fig. 9-13). If a suitable donor site is not located on an adjacent tooth, a free autogenous soft-tissue graft must be used. While the coverage of denuded root surfaces with this method is possible, it is not as favorable as with the pedicle graft. However, the free autogenous soft-tissue graft is effective in creating a zone of attached gingiva at the preoperative level of the alveolar bone. This acts as a good barrier to further recession (see Fig. 9-16).

TREATMENT

The treatment of gingival recession is concerned with halting or at least retarding the progressive loss of tissue and, where possible, restoring gingival heights to cover the exposed root surface. The treatment should include procedures to eliminate as many of the etiological and predisposing factors as possible. A typical sequence of treatment for a patient with gingival recession on the facial surface of a mandibular central incisor (Figs. 9-1 and 9-3) is as follows:

1. Immaculate but nontraumatic plaque control in the involved area must be established. A soft toothbrush directed into the gingival sulcus with a gentle vibratory motion is recommended. The patient should be cautioned to avoid a scrubbing motion with the brush.
2. Scaling and root planing are done if calculus is present and the root surface is rough.
3. Condition of the tissue is reevaluated 6 weeks after the establishment of a good, clean dentogingival environment. If the gingival tissue is pink, firm, clinically uninflamed, and esthetically acceptable and the rate of recession is very slow, no further treatment is needed (Fig. 9-12, C). If the tissue is pink but loose and friable

because the zone of attached gingiva is inadequate, one of the following surgical procedures should be performed to transfer firm, keratinized tissue to the involved area to act as a barrier to further recession:

a. Lateral sliding pedicle flap (Figs. 9-13 and 9-14).
b. Double-papillae flap (Fig. 9-15).
c. Free autogenous soft-tissue graft (Figs. 9-16 and 14-21).
d. Coronally positioned flap. Gingival tissue located just apical to the area of recession is reflected as a full-thickness flap and moved coronally to cover the denuded root surface. A free autogenous soft-tissue graft is frequently required to establish a zone of attached gingiva before performing the repositioning procedure.

When a high frenum or muscle attachment is involved, a frenectomy or detachment of the muscle is done in conjunction with the procedures just mentioned.

The treatment may also include the following when indicated:

1. Root demineralization with citric acid
2. Orthodontic movement or recontouring of the tooth to place it within the alveolar housing
3. Replacement of overcontoured restorations
4. Replacement of prosthetic appliances that impinge on the gingiva
5. Correction of deleterious habits like chewing on pencils or hairpins, which can injure the gingiva
6. Occlusal adjustment

PATIENT EDUCATION

Patients should be informed about areas of recession and the potential problems related to them. Patient cooperation in the treatment of recession is important and should include the correct, gentle use of a soft toothbrush and the elimination of any habits that are injuring the gingival tissues.

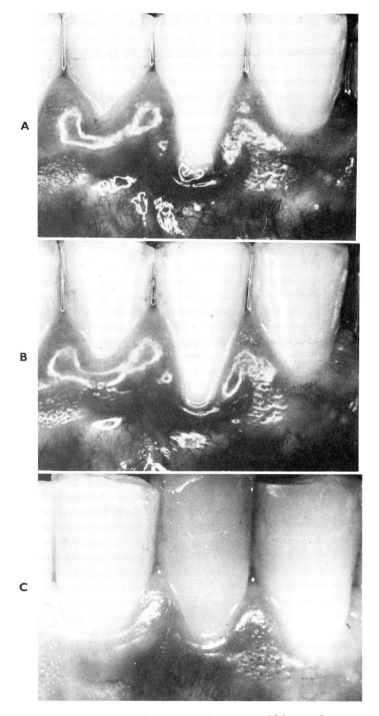

FIGURE 9-12. A, Pretreatment photograph of a 12-year-old boy with apparent gingival recession related to enlargement of adjacent gingiva rather than root exposure. **B,** Three weeks after plaque control scaling and polishing of the teeth. Note the reduction in inflammation and gingival enlargement. **C,** Eighteen months after the initial treatment. Note that the passive eruption (gingival recession) on the adjacent teeth has now reached the same position as that on tooth 24.

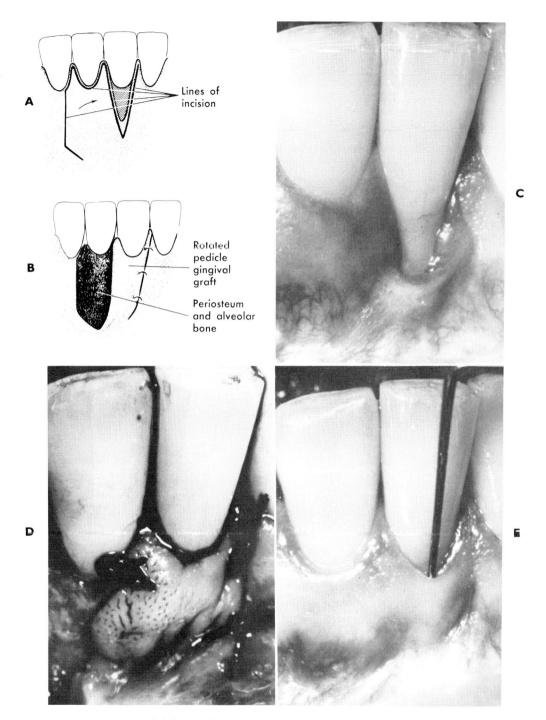

FIGURE 9-13. Lateral sliding pedicle graft technique. **A,** Lines of initial incisions. **B,** Gingiva and contiguous alveolar mucosa on the right central incisor are rotated over onto the exposed root surface on the left central incisor. **C,** Isolated area of gingival recession on the facial surface of tooth 25. Note the wide zone of attached gingiva on tooth 26, which will be the graft donor tissue. The patient is 40 years old. **D,** Clinical surgical procedure in which the gingiva on the facial of tooth 26 has been reflected and repositioned onto the facial surface of tooth 25. **E,** Healing of the graft 3 years after the surgical procedure.

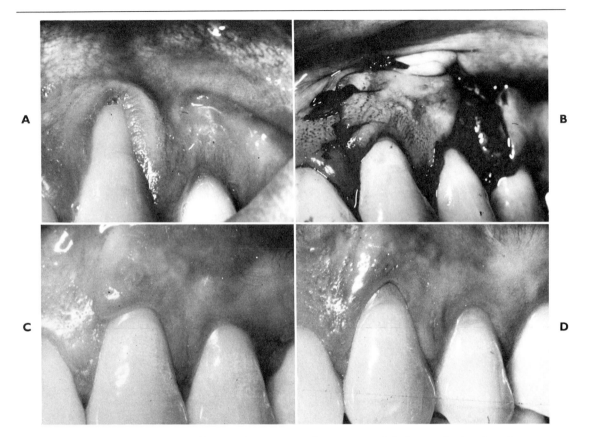

FIGURE 9-14. A, Advanced gingival recession and mucogingival defect on the facial surface of tooth 11 in 21-year-old man. **B,** Lateral sliding pedicle graft moved from the first premolar to the cuspid. **C,** One month following the surgical procedure. **D,** Six years following the surgical procedure. While some recession has recurred, an adequate zone of attached gingiva and considerable root coverage are still present.

PREVENTIVE MEASURES

The methods of preventing gingival recession are somewhat empirical because the exact etiology is often difficult to establish. However, the following procedures aid in controlling many of the factors thought to cause or predispose to gingival recession:

1. Help the patient practice effective nontraumatic plaque control.
2. Treat gingivitis and periodontitis early to prevent tissue destruction and recession.
3. Recommend orthodontic tooth movement when it will help to locate the tooth more within the alveolar housing.
4. Do not do orthodontics in the presence of gingival inflammation or on teeth with inadequate zones of attached gingiva.
5. Treat occlusal trauma when it first appears.
6. Do restorative dentistry in such a way as to minimize gingival injury during the procedure and to create tooth contours that facilitate rather than hinder adequate plaque control.

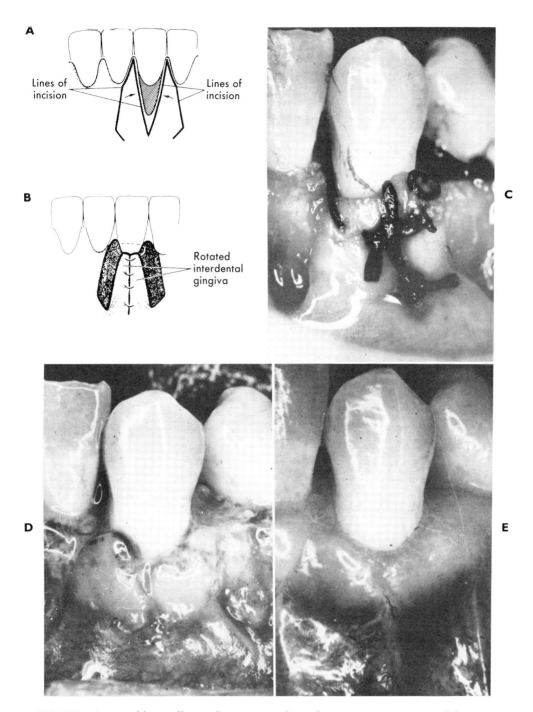

FIGURE 9-15. Double-papillae graft. **A,** Lines of initial incisions. **B,** Diagram of the interdental gingiva and contiguous alveolar mucosa rotated over onto the facial surface of the tooth. **C,** Clinical surgical procedure in which the mesial and distal interdental gingiva has been reflected and repositioned on the facial surface of tooth 22. **D,** Healing of double-papillae graft 1 week after the surgical procedure. **E,** Healing of double-papillae graft 3 years after the surgical procedure.

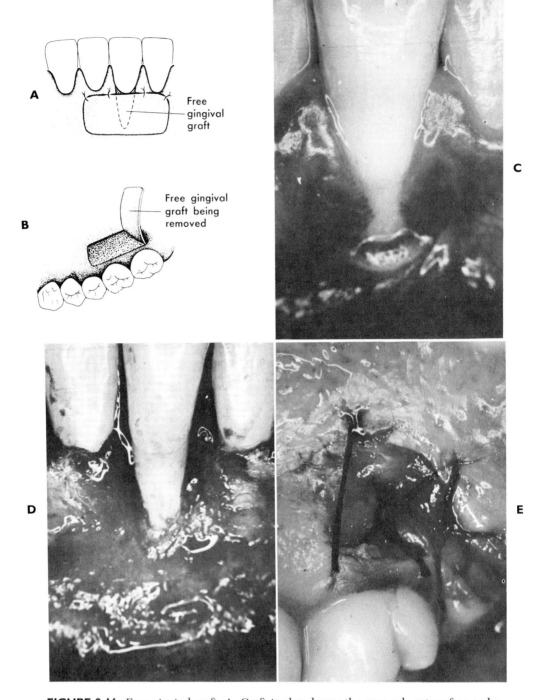

FIGURE 9-16. Free gingival graft. **A,** Graft is placed over the exposed root surface and sutured on its coronal aspects. **B,** Free gingival graft is often obtained from the masticatory mucosa on the palatal surface of the maxillary molars. **C,** Isolated area of recession on the facial surface of tooth 24. **D,** Surgical preparation of the recipient site. The root surface is planed and the epithelium is removed from the alveolar mucosa along with any muscle or loose fibrous attachments. **E,** Donor site. A section of masticatory mucosa was removed from the palatal surface of the maxillary molars.

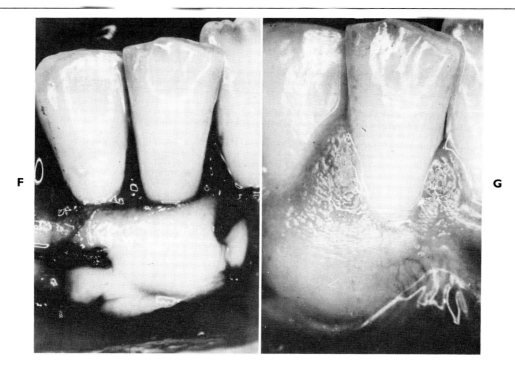

FIGURE 9-16, cont'd. **F,** Graft is placed over the denuded root surface and the surrounding bone. **G,** Healing of the free gingival graft 1 year after the surgical procedure.

7. Design prosthetic appliances so that they do not impinge on the gingival tissues.

SUGGESTED READINGS

Chaikin RW: Elements of surgical treatment in the delivery of periodontal therapy, 1977, Quintessence, Chapter 11.

Hall WB: The current state of mucogingival problems and their therapy, J Periodontol 52:569, 1981.

Holbrook T, and Ochsenbien C: Complete coverage of the denuded root surface with a one stage gingival graft, Int J Periodont Restorative Dent 3:9, 1983.

Maynard JG Jr: Coronal positioning of a previously placed autogenous gingival graft, J Periodontol 48:151, 1977.

Strahan JD, and Waite IM: Color atlas of periodontology, Chicago, 1979, Year Book Medical Publishers, Inc., pp 78-89.

CHAPTER 10
Pericoronitis, Gingival Abscess, Periodontal Abscess, and Cysts

PERICORONITIS
Definition

Pericoronitis is an inflammatory condition of the gingiva and other supporting tissues that surround the crown of a completely or incompletely erupted tooth. It is most commonly found around the mandibular third molars or the mandibular second molars, when they are the most distal tooth in the arch. Pericoronitis can manifest as acute or chronic, depending on the clinical characteristics.

Clinical characteristics

1. Coverage of the occlusal surface of the erupted or partially erupted tooth by a flap of gingival tissue called an *operculum* (formed during tooth eruption) (Fig. 10-1)
2. Swelling and redness of the operculum (Fig. 10-2)
3. Increased tendency to bleed
4. Surface of operculum traumatized and ulcerated
5. Painful and tender area around operculum
6. Purulent exudate in the area caused by the infectious process
7. Limited mandibular movement (trismus)
8. Foul breath
9. Foul taste
10. Possible referred pain to the ear and throat
11. Lymph node inflammatory involvement (lymphadenopathy)
12. Fever
13. Malaise
14. Possible toxic systemic complications

Complications can develop, forming a pericoronal abscess and subsequent space infection and Ludwig's (Vincent's) angina, characterized by swelling of the oropharyngeal area and regional lymph node pathology.

Radiographic signs

In relatively early conditions only soft tissues are involved. Therefore no radiographic changes are seen.

If the condition is left untreated or if complications occur, the infection may spread into the deeper layers of the periodontium and oral tissues. In these situations a diffuse radiolucency may be seen surrounding the coronal aspects of the tooth. A periodontal abscess is a possible sequel of pericoronitis. In this situation damage may occur that will appear on a radiograph.

Histopathology and pathogenesis

Pericoronitis usually appears around teeth that have loosely attached oral mucosa over their occlusal surfaces. The loosely attached operculum creates deep gingival pockets that accumulate plaque and food debris quite readily. The latter initiates gingival inflammation that causes the soft tissues to swell over the occlusal sur-

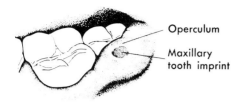

FIGURE 10-1. Pericoronitis on a partially erupted mandibular third molar. The tissue on the occlusal surface is called an operculum. It is being traumatized by the opposing molar. Note imprint of cusp on the operculum.

faces of the teeth. If an opposing tooth is present, it then mechanically traumatizes the inflamed tissue (Fig. 10-1).

The histological picture of these tissues shows acute inflammatory cells, engorged blood vessels, and accumulation of tissue fluids. The inflammatory condition can spread to the adjacent soft tissues, underlying alveolar bone, and peritonsillar tissues and cervical lymph nodes. If not treated, serious complications such as Ludwig's angina, cellulitis, and peritonsillar abscesses can develop.

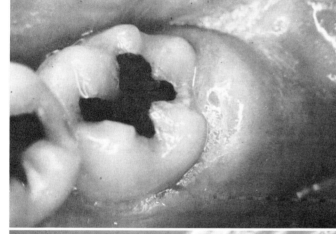

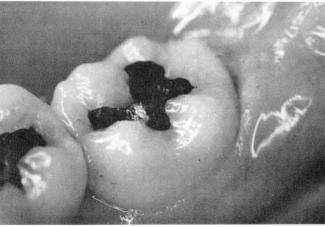

FIGURE 10-2. A, Pericoronitis on the distal aspect of a mandibular third molar. B, Healing 1 week after the scaling and curettage of the affected areas in A.

Etiology

Bacterial plaque, food debris, and mechanical irritation by occlusal forces are the etiological factors responsible for pericoronitis. The space between the operculum and the tooth surface interferes with oral hygiene techniques and is an ideal environment for the accumulation of bacterial plaque and food debris.

The food debris and bacterial accumulation cause inflammation and swelling in the surrounding tissues. When swelling occurs, the operculum becomes mechanically traumatized by the opposing tooth during closure. This swelling aggravates the existing infection.

Nutritional implications

The etiological factors of pericoronitis are local in nature, therefore no nutritional implications are responsible as causative agents.

A diet that is nutritionally adequate, contains no chemically and mechanically irritating foods, and is low in retentive sugars is supportive and recommended in maintaining oral health and resisting infection.

Prognosis

If pericoronitis is treated in its initial stages, the tissues will return to a healthy state. The long-range prognosis for maintaining periodontal health around teeth that have had pericoronitis depends on effective elimination of the operculum and the establishment of a dentogingival environment conducive to effective plaque control. Tooth position and anatomical limitations such as a shallow vestibule or an inadequate arch length often prevent successful surgical intervention. Extraction of such teeth is often necessary to prevent recurrence of the pericoronitis.

If left untreated, pericoronitis can lead to a severe infection with systemic complications as well as progressive destruction of the underlying and surrounding tissues.

Treatment

The treatment of pericoronitis depends on the severity of the condition and the symptoms present.

First appointment

1. Patient history is obtained.
2. Symptoms are examined, a diagnosis is determined, and the extent of involvement is established.
3. Mild, gentle debridement is performed in the space created by the operculum.
   a. Topical anesthetic may be necessary, depending on patient discomfort.
   b. The area can be swabbed with an antiseptic solution.
   c. Extensive curettage and surgical procedures should be avoided at the first appointment.
4. After debridement the area is flushed with warm water.
5. If it becomes necessary to establish drainage, an incision may be made or an iodoform gauze may be inserted under the operculum.
6. Systemic antibiotic therapy is recommended if toxic systemic involvement is noted.
7. The patient is instructed in home care procedures and techniques such as warm salt-water rinses.
8. Depending on the level of discomfort, analgesics may need to be prescribed.

Second appointment (24 to 48 hours after first appointment)

1. Gentle debridement of debris is again performed.
2. The area is then flushed with warm water.
3. The use of the warm saltwater rinses is reinforced.

Third appointment (24 to 48 hours after second appointment)

1. After the infection has subsided, a decision must be made as to whether or not the tooth should be extracted.
2. If the tooth is not extracted, periodontal surgery is often necessary to remove the operculum and create a dentogingival environment conducive to effective plaque control.

Patient education

1. The cause and the mechanism of development of this condition are explained to the patient.
2. The patient is instructed to drink abundant amounts of fluids.
3. Systemic antibiotics may be prescribed and should be taken as directed.
4. To reduce discomfort, the patient should rinse with saltwater hourly—1 teaspoon of salt in a glass of warm water.
5. Patient should perform other oral hygiene techniques—proper brushing, use of antimicrobial mouthwashes, etc.

Preventive measures

Adequate plaque control around erupting teeth and early removal of persistent opercula are the most important preventive measures. Early extraction of an impacted tooth is also a helpful preventive measure.

DENTAL ABSCESSES

A *dental abscess* is a localized, circumscribed, purulent area of inflammation in the tissues surrounding the teeth. The three types of dental abscesses are gingival, periodontal, and periapical.

Dental abscesses may resemble each other from a clinical standpoint, differing only in point of origin and their specific path of infection. The gingival abscess develops through a break in the gingival tissue surface as a result of an acute injury or localized infection of the gingiva; the periodontal abscess develops when the inflammatory drainage from a periodontal pocket is blocked, and the periapical abscess develops from an infection of the pulpal tissue. While the specific abscesses mentioned usually occur alone, they also may exist together.

Gingival abscess
Definition

A gingival abscess is an acute localized inflammatory reaction of the gingiva. It is a response to irritation caused by foreign materials such as toothbrush bristles and toothpicks being forced into the gingiva. It can also develop as a result of food impaction, oral hygiene procedures, dental treatment, or a localized gingival infection.

When the foreign material is forced into the gingiva, it causes a break in the epithelial tissue. Bacteria invade the tissues through this abrasion, causing the localized infectious process. In its beginning stages the abscess appears as a localized area of swelling with a red, smooth, shiny surface. As the lesion progresses, it may become pointed and a purulent exudate may be released from the surface through a fistulous tract.

Gingival abscesses are usually confined to the marginal or interdental gingiva.

The gingival abscess is treatable by an incision to permit drainage, and its prognosis is highly favorable.

Periodontal abscess
Definition

A *periodontal (lateral, parietal) abscess* is a localized, circumscribed purulent area of inflammation in the periodontal tissues. It may be acute or chronic. Acute abscesses often become chronic, and chronic abscesses frequently become acute.

Clinical characteristics (Fig. 10-3)
Acute stage

1. Surrounding gingiva is enlarged, red, edematous, tender, and painful with a smooth, shiny surface.
2. Tooth mobility may be increased.
3. Tooth is sensitive to percussion.
4. Purulent exudate may be discharged from the opening of the pocket.
5. Systemic effects include malaise, fever, and regional lymph node swelling (lymphadenopathy). Face and lips may be swollen.
6. Abscess may appear as a circular elevation (swelling) of the gingiva (Fig. 10-3).
7. Dull, throbbing, radiating pain is present.

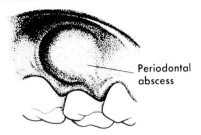

FIGURE 10-3. Periodontal abscess on the buccal surface of a maxillary second premolar.

8. Periodontal pocket is frequently deep and usually communicates with the abscess. This can be noted with a periodontal probe (Fig. 10-4).

Chronic stage. Chronic abscesses are usually asymptomatic, although they frequently advance into the acute stage.

If the abscess has involved both periodontal and peripheral tissues, clinical characteristics and symptoms of both may be present simultaneously.

Radiographic signs

A periodontal abscess usually appears as a radiolucent area lateral to the surface of the root as opposed to the periapical abscess, which typically appears at the apex of the root. However, because of the anatomical location, sometimes no radiographic changes are noted. In the advanced stages of a periodontal abscess extensive bone loss may be noted radiographically.

Radiographs cannot be used as the sole diagnostic aid for periodontal abscesses because of the various locations and stages of development of the abscess.

Histopathology and pathogenesis

Histologically a periodontal abscess appears as a localized accumulation of inflammatory cells circumscribed with a fibrous connective tissue capsule. In the acute abscess the predominant inflammatory cell is the polymorphonuclear leukocyte, and in the chronic situation the

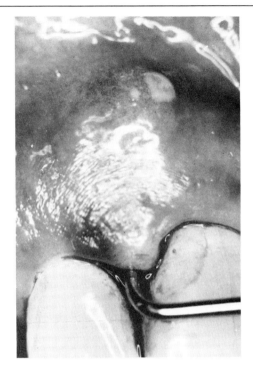

FIGURE 10-4. Periodontal abscess on the mesial aspect of tooth 7. Note that the periodontal probe verifies the communication between the periodontal pocket and the abscess.

principal inflammatory cell is the lymphocyte. Osteoclastic resorption of the surrounding alveolar bone is evident.

Etiology

Periodontal abscesses are associated with periodontal pockets, although these abscesses may occur in the absence of generalized periodontitis.

A periodontal abscess develops when the orifice of the pocket becomes partially or completely blocked. The opening becomes blocked by calculus, plaque, food debris, or foreign objects, making drainage impossible; therefore inflammatory products cannot escape. Bacterial plaque is within the depth of the pocket, and it is the bacterial products that cause irritation and inflammation. Pus, an inflammatory product, cannot drain from the pocket because of the blockage; therefore an abscess occurs.

Certain areas are prone to abscess formation. Bifurcation and trifurcation involvements and deep infrabony pockets are common sites for abscess formation.

Nutritional implications

No specific nutritional etiological factors are associated with abscesses. Patients with diabetes mellitus may be more susceptible to periodontal abscess formation because of a low resistance to infection.

Prognosis

The prognosis of returning a tooth that has a periodontal abscess to periodontal health depends on the amount and type of bone loss, the position of the tooth and abscess, and the mobility of the tooth.

The prognosis for bone regeneration following an acute infection is much better than bone regeneration following a chronic lesion.

Treatment

1. Proper diagnosis is important because periodontal abscesses may be misdiagnosed as periapical abscesses and therefore mistreated. Proper diagnosis depends on clinical findings, radiographic findings, and pulp testing.
2. First step is reduction of the abscess and the acute inflammation. Drainage should be established by curetting the pocket or incising the abscess. Extracting the tooth when necessary will also provide drainage of the purulent exudate.
3. Antibiotic therapy is indicated when fever or cervical lymphadenopathy is present.
4. Second step is reduction of the pocket to remove the cause of the abscess. This can usually be accomplished most efficiently with periodontal flap surgery.
5. Occlusal adjustment or temporary splinting may be necessary.

6. If the abscess has involved the periodontal tissues surrounding the apex of the root, endodontic as well as periodontal treatment will be necessary to allow healing to take place.

Patient education

1. The cause and the mechanism of this condition should be explained to the patient.
2. The patient is instructed to drink abundant amounts of fluids.
3. Systemic antibiotics may be prescribed and should be taken as directed.
4. The patient should rinse with hot water every 2 hours if prescribed.

Preventive measures

1. Diabetic patients with periodontitis should receive early definitive medical and periodontal therapy because they are particularly susceptible to developing periodontal abscesses.
2. Patients with periodontal pockets or potential periodontal pockets should be closely observed and placed on a rigid plaque control program and recall policy.
3. Effective pocket reduction and relief of occlusal trauma should be performed.

CYSTS

A *cyst* is a sac that contains fluid. Two types of cysts appear in the periodontium: gingival cysts and periodontal cysts.

The *gingival cyst*, if it becomes clinically noticeable, appears as a bluish gray localized enlargement. It is nodular in appearance and resembles a mucocele. Such a cyst is painless and can involve either the attached or the marginal gingiva. Gingival cysts are not most commonly located on the lingual surface in the mandibular canine and premolar area. Because they usually involve only the soft tissue no radiographic findings are seen. If removal is indicated, the prognosis is favorable.

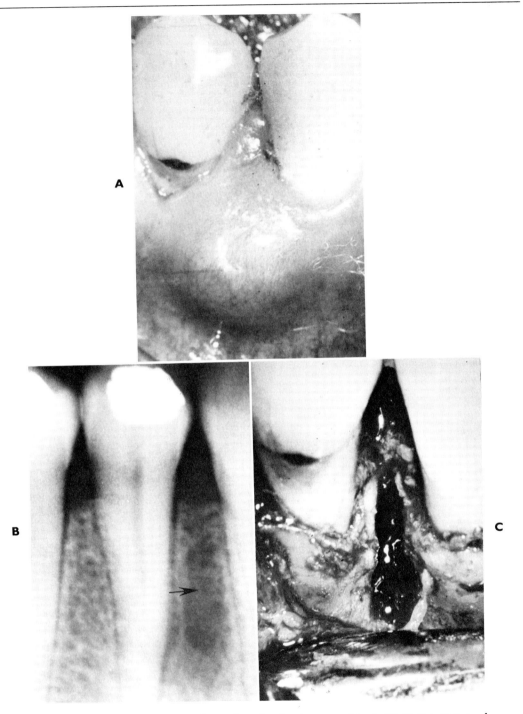

FIGURE 10-5. **A,** Periodontal cyst located on the distal aspect of tooth 27. **B,** Interproximal radiolucent image of the periodontal cyst *(arrow).* **C,** Interproximal bone defect noted during the surgical removal of the cyst.

Histologically the gingival cyst appears as a localized hollow space within the connective tissue of the gingiva lined with stratified squamous epithelium.

A *periodontal cyst* radiographically resembles a periodontal abscess. Both appear adjacent to the lateral surface of the root as a radiolucent lesion bordered by a radiopaque line. A periodontal cyst usually appears asymptomatic, although localized gingival swelling may be present. Periodontal cysts produce destruction of the periodontal tissues in the surrounding area. Like the gingival cyst, the periodontal cyst most commonly occurs in the mandibular canine and premolar areas (Fig. 10-5).

Both gingival and periodontal cysts are believed to develop from odontogenic epithelium in the periodontal ligament or the gingiva. If the cysts become infected, they often form abscesses.

Histologically the periodontal cyst appears as a hollow space adjacent to the lateral surface of the root of a tooth lined with epithelium. Osteoclastic bone resorption may be evident in the bone surrounding the cyst.

SUGGESTED READINGS

Baer PN, and Morris M: Textbook of periodontics, Philadelphia, 1977, JB Lippincott Co, pp 307-310.

Carranza F: Glickman's clinical periodontology, ed 5, Philadelphia, 1979, WB Saunders Co, pp 273-274, 688-695.

Schluger S, Yuodelis R, and Page R: Periodontal disease, Philadelphia, 1977, Lea & Febiger, pp 240-242.

Strahan JD, and Waite IM: Color atlas of periodontology, Chicago, 1979, Year Book Medical Publishers, Inc., pp 37-39.

CHAPTER II
Periodontal Examination, Diagnosis, Prognosis, and Treatment Plan

PERIODONTAL EXAMINATION

The periodontal examination is that portion of the comprehensive oral evaluation that deals specifically with the periodontal tissues. The objectives of this procedure are to determine the following:

1. Whether the patient's periodontium is healthy or diseased
2. The activity and extent of the tissue damage if pathological changes are present
3. Characteristics of the patient's disease that determine the diagnosis, etiology, prognosis, and treatment plan

The procedures performed to evaluate the periodontium can be divided into two main categories:

1. Patient's chief complaint and the medical and dental history
2. Physical and radiographic evaluation:
   a. Vital signs and general health appearance
   b. Extraoral head and neck findings
   c. Intraoral head and neck findings

Patient's chief complaint and the medical and dental history

The *chief complaint* is "the principal reason that the patient has sought a dental examination and/or treatment."

While the patient's reason for seeking dental treatment is not always the most urgent need, it is important for the examiner to assess the patient's principal concern and try to satisfy this desire through emergency treatment or by an adequate explanation of the nature of the problem and why it cannot be corrected immediately. Demonstrating empathy for the patient's expectations during the initial visit helps stimulate patient cooperation and successful comprehensive treatment.

The *medical history* is an assessment of the patient's general body health as evaluated by the patient. The patient is asked a series of questions to obtain the necessary information. Standardized questions have been developed for this purpose and are available in printed forms. One example is the health questionnaire prepared by the American Dental Association (Fig. 11-1). However, flexibility and individuality are encouraged when taking the history. The following list of principal areas to cover can be used as a guide in developing questions:

1. Date history is taken
2. Patient identification information including name, address, telephone number, occupation, marital status, sex, and age
3. General health and date of last physical examination
4. Current treatment and any medications being taken at this time
5. Name and address of physician
6. History of serious illness or operations
7. Diet and nutrition
8. Allergies
   a. Local anesthetics
   b. Penicillin
   c. Others

Medical History

Date _____

Name _____ _____ _____   Address _____
　　　Last　　　　　　First　　　　　　Middle　　　　　Number, Street

City _____ State _____   Zip Code _____   Home _____   Business _____
　　　　　　　　　　　　　　　　　　　　　　　　　　　　　　　　　　Phone　　　　　　Phone

Date of Birth _____ Sex _____ Height _____ Weight _____ Occupation _____

Social Security No. _____   Single _____ Married _____ Name of Spouse _____

Closest Relative _____   Phone _____

If you are completing this form for another person, what is your relationship to that person? _____

Referred by _____

In the following questions, circle yes or no, whichever applies. Your answers are for our records only and will be considered confidential.

1. Are you in good health? . . . . Yes　No
2. Has there been any change in your general health within the past year? . . . . Yes　No
3. My last physical examination was on _____
4. Are you now under the care of a physician? . . . . Yes　No
   If so, what is the condition being treated? _____
5. The name and address of my physician is _____
   _____
   _____
6. Have you had any serious illness or operation? . . . . Yes　No
   If so, what was the illness or operation? _____
7. Have you been hospitalized or had a serious illness within the past five (5) years? . . . . . . Yes　No
   If so, what was the problem? _____
8. Do you have or have you had any of the following diseases or problems?
   a. Damaged heart valves or artificial heart valves, including heart murmur . . . . Yes　No
   b. Congenital heart lesions . . . . Yes　No
   c. Cardiovascular disease (heart trouble, heart attack, coronary insufficiency, coronary occlusion, high blood pressure,
      arteriosclerosis, stroke) . . . . Yes　No
      1. Do you have pain in chest upon exertion? . . . . Yes　No
      2. Are you ever short of breath after mild exercise? . . . . Yes　No
      3. Do your ankles swell? . . . . Yes　No
      4. Do you get short of breath when you lie down, or do you require extra pillows when you sleep? . . . . Yes　No
      5. Do you have a cardiac pacemaker? . . . . Yes　No
   d. Allergy . . . . Yes　No
   e. Sinus trouble . . . . Yes　No
   f. Asthma or hay fever . . . . Yes　No
   g. Hives or a skin rash . . . . Yes　No
   h. Fainting spells or seizures . . . . Yes　No
   i. Diabetes . . . . Yes　No
      1. Do you have to urinate (pass water) more than six times a day? . . . . Yes　No
      2. Are you thirsty much of the time? . . . . Yes　No
      3. Does your mouth frequently become dry? . . . . Yes　No
   j. Hepatitis, jaundice or liver disease . . . . Yes　No
   k. Arthritis . . . . Yes　No
   l. Inflammatory rheumatism (painful swollen joints) . . . . Yes　No
   m. Stomach ulcers . . . . Yes　No
   n. Kidney trouble . . . . Yes　No
   o. Tuberculosis . . . . Yes　No
   p. Do you have a persistent cough or cough up blood? . . . . Yes　No
   q. Low blood pressure . . . . Yes　No
   r. Venereal disease . . . . Yes　No
   s. Epilepsy . . . . Yes　No
   t. Psychiatric problems . . . . Yes　No
   u. Cancer . . . . Yes　No
   v. AIDS or other immunosuppressive disorders . . . . Yes　No
   w. Other _____

B500　　　　　　　　　　　　　　　　　(over)

FIGURE 11-1. Health questionnaire prepared by the American Dental Association (Copyright by the American Dental Association. Reprinted with permission). *Continued.*

9. Have you had abnormal bleeding associated with previous extractions, surgery, or trauma? . . . . Yes No
   a. Do you bruise easily? . . . . Yes No
   b. Have you ever required a blood transfusion? . . . . Yes No
     If so, explain the circumstances _____

10. Do you have any blood disorder such as anemia? . . . . Yes No

11. Have you had surgery, x-ray or drug treatment for a tumor, growth, or other condition of your head or neck? . . . . . . Yes No

12. Are you taking any drug or medicine?. . . . . Yes No
   If so, what? _____

13. Are you taking any of the following:
   a. Antibiotics or sulfa drugs . . . . Yes No
   b. Anticoagulants (blood thinners) . . . . Yes No
   c. Medicine for high blood pressure . . . . Yes No
   d. Cortisone (steroids). . . . . Yes No
   e. Tranquilizers . . . . Yes No
   f. Antihistamines . . . . Yes No
   g. Aspirin . . . . Yes No
   h. Insulin, tolbutamide (Orinase) or similar drug. . . . . Yes No
   i. Digitalis or drugs for heart trouble . . . . Yes No
   j. Nitroglycerin . . . . Yes No
   k. Oral contraceptive or other hormonal therapy . . . . Yes No
   l. Other _____

14. Are you allergic or have you reacted adversely to:
   a. Local anesthetics . . . . Yes No
   b. Penicillin or other antibiotics. . . . . Yes No
   c. Sulfa drugs . . . . Yes No
   d. Barbiturates, sedatives, or sleeping pills . . . . Yes No
   e. Aspirin . . . . Yes No
   f. Iodine. . . . . Yes No
   g. Codeine or other narcotics . . . . Yes No
   h. Other _____

15. Have you had any serious trouble associated with any previous dental treatment? . . . . Yes No
   If so, explain _____

16. Do you have any disease, condition, or problem not listed above that you think I should know about? . . . . Yes No
   If so, explain _____

17. Are you employed in any situation which exposes you regularly to x-rays or other ionizing radiation? . . . . Yes No

18. Are you wearing contact lenses? . . . . Yes No

19. Have you had anything to eat or drink in the last 4 hours?. . . . . Yes No

20. Are you wearing removable dental appliances? . . . . Yes No

Women

21. Are you pregnant? . . . . Yes No

22. Do you have any problems associated with your menstrual period?. . . . . Yes No

23. Are you nursing? . . . . Yes No

Chief Dental Complaint

I certify that I have read and understand the above. I acknowledge that my questions, if any, about the inquiries set forth above have been answered to my satisfaction. I will not hold my dentist, or any other member of his/her staff, responsible for any errors or omissions that I may have made in the completion of this form.

_____
Signature of Patient

American Dental Association

_____
Signature of Dentist

FIGURE 11-1, cont'd

9. Cardiovascular system
    a. History of rheumatic fever
    b. Blood pressure
    c. Pulse rate
    d. History of cardiovascular insufficiency
    e. Other
10. Blood dyscrasias
    a. Abnormal bleeding or clotting times
    b. Abnormal cellular counts
    c. Other disorders
11. Respiratory system disorders
12. Gastrointestinal system disorders
13. Genitourinary system disorders of females
    a. Pregnancy
    b. Contraceptive medications
14. Neurological disorders
15. Dermatological disorders
16. Psychological disorders
17. Infectious diseases

The purposes of assessing a patient's general body health as part of a periodontal examination are to alert the examiner to the following:

1. Information that might help determine if systemic etiologic factors are present that can affect gingival or periodontal tissue changes—example: diabetes mellitus, blood dyscrasias, and the drug phenytoin for epilepsy
2. Medical disorders that will modify the type of periodontal treatment to be rendered—example: history of rheumatic heart disease requiring antibiotic premedication before any periodontal instrumentation
3. Contagious disorders that might endanger the health of the examiner or other staff members—examples: venereal disease, AIDS.

Positive findings in any of these categories indicate the need for consultation with an appropriate physician. Diagnostic laboratory procedures may be indicated and should be ordered and evaluated in conjunction with the patient's physician.

The *dental history* consists of a series of questions that will help the examiner determine the patient's attitude toward dental health and the response to previous dental treatment. Following are the principal categories to evaluate:

1. Patient's attitude toward dental health
2. Date and nature of last dental treatment
3. Regularity of previous dental treatment
4. Oral hygiene habits
    a. Toothbrush—type and frequency
    b. Dental floss—type and frequency
    c. Toothpicks
    d. Mouthrinses
    e. Other aids
5. History of and response to previous major dental treatment
    a. Preventive treatments
    b. Periodontics
    c. Restorations
    d. Prostheses
    e. Endodontic therapy
    f. Orthodontics
    g. Oral surgery
    h. Other
6. Habits related to oral health or disease
    a. Bruxism
    b. Clenching
    c. Smoking
    d. Other
7. History of myofacial pain dysfunction syndrome

Physical and radiographic evaluation
Vital signs and general health appearance

Evaluating a patient's general health enables the operator to be as confident as possible that the patient will not be endangered during dental treatment. In addition, the dental profession has the opportunity to provide a valuable health detection service because, in general, more people see the dentist on a regular basis than a physician. A blood pressure determination at regular dental visits to note signs of hypertension is an example of such a service.

Following are the *vital signs* to be included in the examination:

1. Blood pressure. Normal values vary according to age.
   a. Children 6 to 10 years old: 70 to 90 mm Hg/50 to 70 mm Hg
   b. Adolescents and young adults: 120 mm Hg/80 mm Hg
   c. Middle age: 120 to 140 mm Hg/70 to 80 mm Hg
   d. Older age: 140 to 160 mm Hg/90 to 100 mm Hg
   e. Guidelines for adults. The guidelines set forth by the American Heart Association for adult blood pressure are as follows:
      (1) 138 mm Hg/88 mm Hg and lower = normal
      (2) 140 mm Hg/90 mm Hg to 158 mm Hg/94 mm Hg = borderline
      (3) 160 mm Hg/95 mm Hg and higher = elevated
      (4) 180 mm Hg/110 mm Hg and higher = immediate referral
2. Pulse rate. Normal range is 60 to 80 beats per minute.
3. Respiration rate. Normal range at rest is 12 to 16 respiratory movements per minute.
4. Body temperature. 98.6° F.

Following are the *general health appearance* factors to note:

1. General patient color: jaundiced, cyanotic, pallor, flush, etc.
2. Ease of respiration
3. Walking gait
4. Body weight and contours
5. Extremities: control of movement, edema, ulcerations

Extraoral head and neck findings

The extraoral findings include the following:

1. Cervical lymphadenopathy
2. Abnormal external contours: swellings, enlargements, defects
3. Abnormal skin elevations, ulcerations, or colors

4. Eyes: exophthalmos, color, dilated pupils, etc.

Intraoral head and neck findings

The intraoral findings as they relate to the periodontal portion of the examination should be noted to adequately determine the following:

1. Presence of periodontal disease
2. Activity and extent of periodontal destruction
3. Etiology of periodontal disease
4. Periodontal diagnosis
5. Periodontal prognosis
6. Periodontal treatment plan

The last three will be discussed later.

Presence of periodontal disease. Initial evaluations can help determine the presence or absence of periodontal disease or other intraoral soft-tissue pathological changes.

Evaluate the color, contour, consistency, and size of the oral mucosa, lips, tongue, oropharynx, floor of the mouth, and soft palate.

Evaluate the gingiva according to the following criteria (note the *generalized* appearance of the gingival tissues as well as any *localized* changes that deviate from those seen throughout the mouth):

1. Color: pink, red, bluish red, or other color variations
2. Consistency: normal, edematous, fibrotic, fibroedematous
3. Texture (stippling): normal, decreased, increased
4. Contour (both marginal and papillary): normal, rounded, cratered, or other anatomical aberrations
5. Size: normal, increased, decreased
6. Position: adjacent to cementoenamel junction, receded, coronal to cementoenamel junction
7. Bleeding or exudate on probing: no or yes, slight, moderate, or severe
8. Width of attached gingiva
   a. Adequate in all areas
   b. Inadequate in localized areas (mucogingival defects)

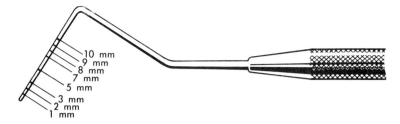

FIGURE 11-2. University of Michigan "O" periodontal probe with Williams Markings.

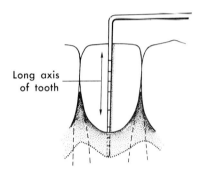

FIGURE 11-3. Correct use of a periodontal probe to measure the depth of the gingival sulcus on the facial surface of a tooth. Note that the probe is held parallel to the long axis of the tooth. It is recording a depth of 2.5 mm.

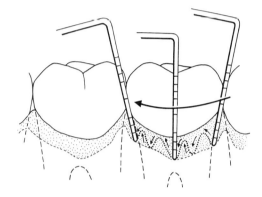

FIGURE 11-4. Periodontal probe is moved through the gingival sulcus, and the deepest point in each area is recorded. The probes have to be slightly tilted off the long axis of the tooth to keep the tip of the probe in contact with the tooth surface being evaluated.

(1) Type I: keratinized gingiva present, but the probing depth extends to or beyond the mucogingival junction (Fig. 11-14, *A*)

(2) Type II: no keratinized gingiva (Fig. 11-14, *B*); high frenum or muscle attachment often present

Extent of periodontal destruction

Evaluation of probing depths. Use a thin calibrated periodontal probe (Fig. 11-2) to determine the depth and topography of the gingival sulci periodontal pockets, and attachment levels. Because the gingival tissues often appear pink, firm, and healthy even though advanced periodontitis is present, it is necessary to carefully probe each gingival sulcus or pocket to determine the presence of the disease. A periodontal examination is not complete unless it includes a recording and an evaluation of the probing depths. The following technique is recommended to determine the clinical probing depths on all surfaces of each tooth. The measurement should determine in millimeters the distance between the most apical point on the tooth reached by the tip of the probe and the crest of the marginal gingiva.

1. Insert the periodontal probe as parallel with the long axis of the tooth as possible but keeping the tip of the probe in contact with the tooth until firm resistance is met (Figs. 11-3 and 11-4).

2. Begin on the distal surface of the most posterior tooth in either the maxillary or mandibular arch and walk the probe mesially through the pockets along the fa-

cial, interproximal, and lingual surfaces of each tooth (Fig. 11-4). Record three measurements from the facial aspect and three measurements from the lingual aspect of each tooth. Use a chart with adequate space to clearly note the probing depths (Fig. 11-5). The measurements are determined in millimeters and represent the deepest points on the following surfaces:

a. Distal surfaces as determined from the facial aspects of the teeth (slight angulation of the probe is often required to reach the deepest point apical to the interproximal contact areas) (Fig. 11-6, *A* and *B*)
b. Facial surfaces (Fig. 11-4)
c. Mesial surfaces as determined from the facial aspects of the teeth
d. Distal surfaces as determined from the lingual (palatal) aspects of the teeth (Fig. 11-6, *C*)
e. Lingual (palatal) surfaces
f. Mesial surfaces as determined from the lingual (palatal) aspects of the teeth

Because of the presence of interproximal contact areas, it is sometimes necessary to tilt the periodontal probe slightly to reach the most apical depth of interproximal pockets (Fig. 11-6). It is more important to identify the level of the tissue attachment than to maintain the probe parallel to the long axis of the tooth. When using the probe, the operator should attempt to keep the tip of the probe in contact with the tooth and not to penetrate the soft tissue wall of the pocket (Fig. 11-7).

Recent studies have shown that the forces commonly generated by clinicians when using the periodontal probe result in determining the level of the healthy gingival fiber attachment rather than the coronal level of the junctional epithelium attachment (actual gingival sulcus or pocket depth) (Fig. 11-8). The more inflamed the tissues the greater is the chance of penetrating the junctional epithelium and recording probing depths (connective tissue at-

tachment levels) in excess of the actual pocket depths (junctional epithelium attachment level). The recognition of this discrepancy in probing has resulted in the current use of the term *probing depths* rather than *pocket depths* when referring to periodontal probing measurements. However, the clinician should avoid excessive pressures and abrupt movements, which cause perforations of the sulcular and junctional epithelia, inaccurate pocket depth determinations, and undue patient discomfort. Newly designed pressure-sensitive and electronic probes are now available to minimize these difficulties.

The operator must also be careful to probe apical to calculus accumulations. A large subgingival deposit can create a ledge that will prevent the probe from reaching the most apical level of the pocket unless the probe is moved laterally and beyond the calculus (Fig. 11-9).

Other evaluations. In addition to the probing depths, the periodontal probe is used to determine the extent of the periodontal tissue destruction by measuring the distance between the level of the junctional epithelial attachments and the cementoenamel junctions (gingival attachment levels). There is a consistent 1 to 2 mm distance between the points on the tooth where the junctional epithelium and the periodontal ligament are attached. Therefore a determination of the gingival attachment level also indicates the bone and periodontal ligament attachment levels at a slightly apical position on the tooth. Gingival attachment level measurements are made by determining with a periodontal probe the distance between the level of the junctional epithelium and the cementoenamel junction or some other fixed reference point on the tooth. If the marginal gingiva has receded apical to the cementoenamel junction, the measurement is visualized by noting the distance between the most apical position of the tip of the periodontal probe when inserted into the sulcus or pocket and the cementoenamel junction (Fig. 11-10, *A*). How-

Text continued on p. 134.

Missing Teeth — X	Exist. Gold — Diagonal Line	Mobility — N-1,2,3	Pulpal Response:
Impacted Teeth — Circle	" Non-Metal — Outline	Osseous Defect — OD	I — Ice
Caries — Outline in Red	Open Contact — //	Muco-Ging. Defect — MG	H — Heat
Decalcification — ✳	Defective Contact — }{	Furcation Invol. — Outline	E — Electric
Periapical Path. — ᗡ	Food Impaction — ↓	Fixed Appliance — ⟅⟆	P — Percussion
Defective Rest. — Def.→	Gingival Line — ～	Drifted, extruded, rotated →	
Exist. Amal. — Solid	Perio. Pocket — in red ( )	Exist. Endo. Treatment — Darken Canal	
		Pulpotomy (PQ) or Pulp Capping (PC)	

Tooth Number	1	2	3	4	5	6	7	8	9	10	11	12	13	14	15	16
Probing Depths-F		423	525	323	323	3/2	2/2	2/2	2/2	2/2	2/3	4/3	314	524	323	
Mobility		N	I	I	N	N	N	I	I	N	N	N	N	N	N	
Pulpal Response																

RIGHT   LEFT

Tooth Number	1	2	3	4	5	6	7	8	9	10	11	12	13	14	15	16
Probing Depths-L		423	425	423	313	2/2	2/2	2/2	2/2	2/2	2/2	313	313	423	323	

Tooth Number	32	31	30	29	28	27	26	25	24	23	22	21	20	19	18	17
Probing Depths-L		423	313	423	433	3/2	2/3	2/2	2/2	2/2	2/3	323	323	523	333	

RIGHT   LEFT

Tooth Number	32	31	30	29	28	27	26	25	24	23	22	21	20	19	18	17
Probing Depths-F		523	323	323	323	3/2	2/2	323	313	2/3	313	323	324	423	324	
Mobility		N	2	I	I	N	N	I	I	I	N	N	N	N	N	
Pulpal Response																

Static: **OCCLUSAL ANALYSIS** Functional:

Angle's Class_____
Overbite_____
Overjet_____
Curve of spee_____
Crossbite_____
Vertical dimension_____
Free-way space_____
Wear Facets_____
Other_____

Centric Prematurities   YES   NO
If so locate initial contact_____
Excursive Interferences (locate)

	Working		**Balancing**
RL	_____		_____
LL	_____		_____
Prot.	_____		_____
Habits	_____		

PREVENTION		
	1st visit	recall
Date		
PHP		
GI		
DMF-S		
INST.		

Signs of TMJ Disorders:
Mandibular deviation_____
Limited opening or hypermobility
TMJ area: tenderness, clicking, crepitus

FIGURE 11-5. Dental chart with adequate space to record probing depth measurements and tooth mobility determinations.   *Continued.*

PERIODONTAL FINDINGS

Gingiva: Describe whether changes are generalized or localized - if localized, specify where.

Color:	Tooth positions contributing to disease:
Consistency:	
Texture:	Iatrogenic etiologic factors:
Contour:	
Size:	Diagnosis:
Position:	
	Etiology:
Bleeding upon probing or exudation:	
Width of attached gingiva:	
Average probing depths and types:	Prognosis:
Muco-gingival defects:	
Furcation involvements:	

PERIODONTAL CASE TYPES

Case Type I - Gingivitis - Gingival pockets, no bone loss.

Case Type II - Early Periodontitis - moderate periodontal pockets, early bone loss.

Case Type III - Moderate Periodontitis - moderate to deep periodontal pockets, moderate to severe bone loss, tooth mobility.

Case Type IV - Advanced Periodontitis - severe destruction of periodontal structures with increased tooth mobility.

Comments:

FIGURE 11-5, cont'd

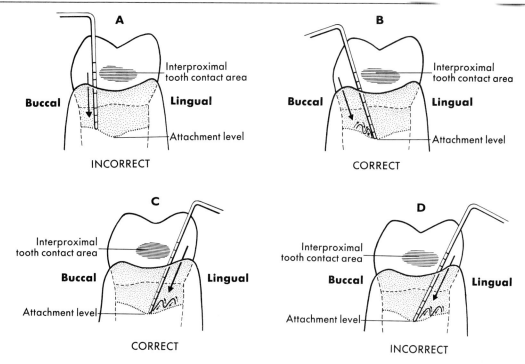

FIGURE 11-6. Probing interproximal tooth surfaces. **A,** If a probe is kept parallel to the long axis of the tooth, the deepest point of the attachment level is often not reached because the interproximal contact area prevents the parallel insertion of the probe along the entire interproximal tooth surface. **B,** Slight angulation and stepping of the probe apical to the contact area and to the deepest attachment level as determined from the buccal aspect of the teeth. **C,** View **B** from the lingual aspect of the tooth. **D,** Avoid excessive angulation, which will indicate exaggerated probing depths.

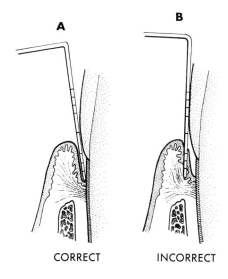

FIGURE 11-7. Use of periodontal probe. **A,** Correct placement of probe keeping tip in contact with the tooth. **B,** Incorrect placement of probe and soft tissue perforation.

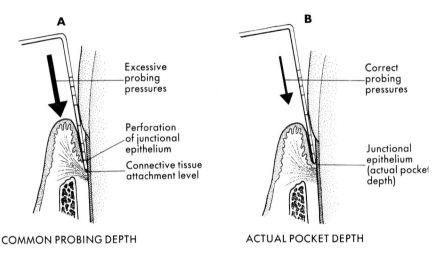

FIGURE 11-8. **A**, Common probing depth. Note perforation of junctional epithelium and determination of connective tissue attachment level rather than actual pocket depth. **B**, Actual pocket depth. Note more accurate determination of actual pocket depth with firm but not excessive probing pressures.

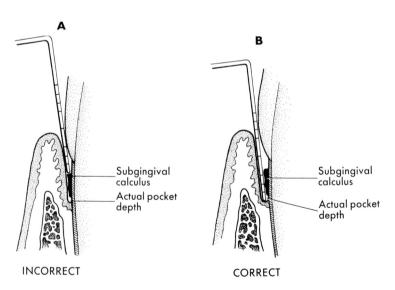

FIGURE 11-9. **A**, Incorrect probing depth indicated because of ledge of subgingival calculus. **B**, Correct probing depth determined by lateral and apical movement of the probe around the calculus deposit.

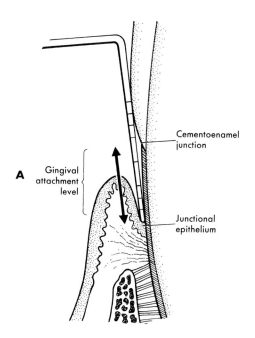

A

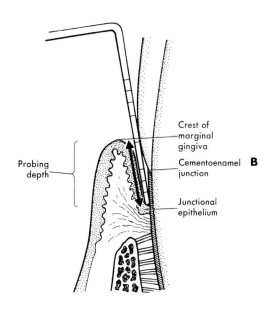

B

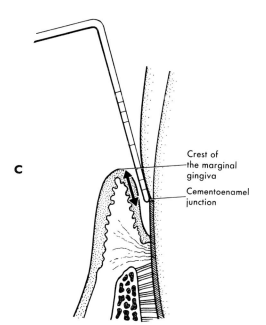

C

FIGURE 11-10. Determining gingival attachment levels. If the cementoenamel junction is exposed, measure the distance between the most apical position of the tip of the probe and the cementoenamel junction, **A.** If the cementoenamel junction is not exposed, measure the probing depth, **B,** and then measure the distance from the crest of the marginal gingiva to the cementoenamel junction, **C.** The probing depth minus the distance from the crest of the gingiva to the cementoenamel junction equals the gingival attachment level.

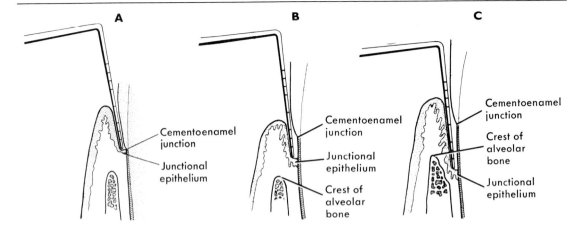

FIGURE 11-11. **A,** Gingival pocket. The periodontal probe can only penetrate to the cementoenamel junction. **B,** Suprabony periodontal pocket. The periodontal probe should penetrate beyond the cementoenamel junction but not pass apical to the crest of the alveolar bone. **C,** Infrabony periodontal pocket. The periodontal probe should penetrate beyond the cementoenamel junction and pass apical to the crest of the alveolar bone.

ever, if the crest of the marginal gingiva is coronal to the cementoenamel junction, the following method must be used to determine the gingival attachment level:

1. Measure the probing depth (Fig. 11-10, *B*).
2. Measure the distance from the crest of the marginal gingiva to the cementoenamel junction (Fig. 11-10, *C*).
3. The probing depth minus the distance from the crest of the gingiva to the cementoenamel junction equals the gingival attachment level.

Determining the gingival attachment levels on a regular basis is a way to evaluate the stability or progressing destruction of the periodontal tissues. In periodontal research the gingival attachment level measurements are considered to be more reflective of the periodontal status than is the probing depth.

The periodontal probe is also used to determine the topography and classification of periodontal pockets. Using the tip of the probe to explore the root surface and the variation in the attachment levels can help visualize the to-

pography of a pocket. The following criteria are used to determine the pocket classification.

1. Gingival pockets (Fig. 11-11, *A*). The periodontal probe should not penetrate apically beyond the cementoenamel junction.
2. Suprabony periodontal pockets (Fig. 11-11, *B*). The periodontal probe should penetrate beyond the cementoenamel junction but not pass apical to the crest of the alveolar bone.
3. Infrabony periodontal pockets (Fig. 11-11, *C*). The periodontal probe should penetrate beyond the cementoenamel junction and pass apical to the crest of the adjacent alveolar bone.

Furcation involvements. The presence of furcation involvements is detected most effectively by the periodontal probe. If the periodontitis has progressed to the extent that it has destroyed the periodontium in the furcations of the posterior teeth, the periodontal probe can be passed directly into the furcation spaces. The straight periodontal probe is sometimes adequate to detect facial and lin-

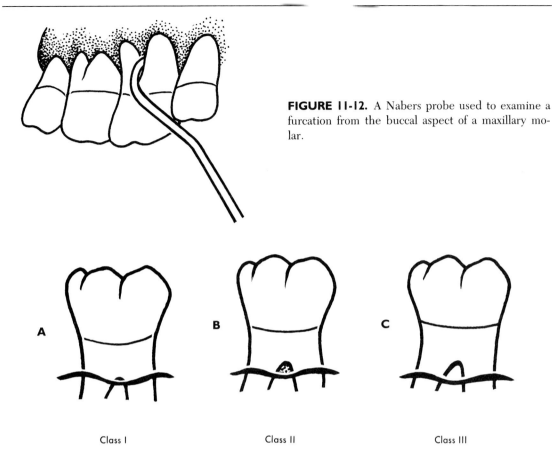

FIGURE 11-12. A Nabers probe used to examine a furcation from the buccal aspect of a maxillary molar.

Class I   Class II   Class III

FIGURE 11-13. Classification of furcations. **A,** Class I: 1 to 2 mm horizontal penetration of probe into furcation. **B,** Class II: More than 1 to 2 mm of horizontal penetration of the probe but not completely through the root. **C,** Class III: Penetration of the probe completely through the furcation to the opposite side of the tooth.

gual furcation involvements. However, special curved probes (Nabers-1 and Nabers-2) are helpful in determining the presence and depths of furcation defects particularly (Fig. 11-12).

Furcations are classified as follows (Fig. 11-13):

Class I   This is the early stage and indicates a suprabony pocket with minimal bone resorption in the furcation. The probe enters the furcation horizontally approximately 1 or 2 mm, and the arch of the furcation can be detected (Fig. 11-13, A).

Class II   The bone resorption extends farther into the furcation but not completely through it. The probe penetrates more than 1 or 2 mm horizontally into the furcation (Fig. 11-13, B)

Class III   The bone resorption extends completely through the furcation. This allows the probe to penetrate from one surface of a tooth to another through the furcation (Fig. 11-13, C).

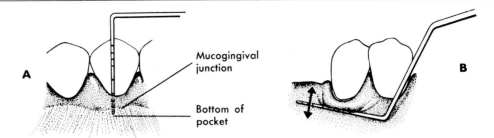

FIGURE 11-14. Determination of adequate zones of attached gingiva or mucogingival defects. **A,** If the periodontal probe passes into the gingival sulcus (pocket) to or beyond the mucogingival junction, there is a lack of attached gingiva. Type I mucogingival defect. **B,** If the marginal gingiva moves when the periodontal probe is activated, usually no attached gingiva is present. Type II mucogingival defect.

Mucogingival defects. Mucogingival defects should be identified according to the following guidelines:

1. When the periodontal probe penetrates into the sulcus or pocket to or beyond the mucogingival junction, the lack of attached gingiva is called a mucogingival defect.

2. If the marginal tissue appears firm in consistency and covered with keratinized epithelium, it is classified as a Type I mucogingival defect. (Figs. 11-14, *A,* and 14-2, *B*).

3. If the marginal tissue appears soft in consistency, is covered with a thin, nonkeratinized epithelium, and is only loosely attached to underlying structures, it is classified as a Type II mucogingival defect. This type of defect is identified if the marginal gingiva moves when a periodontal probe is placed horizontally on the marginal tissue and moved apicocoronally. In this situation the alveolar mucosa creates the marginal tissue (Figs. 11-14, *B,* and 14-2, *D*).

Tooth mobility. Using the handles of two dental instruments, apply alternate pressures on the facial and lingual surfaces of each tooth (Fig. 11-15). The mobility is graded according to the following criteria:

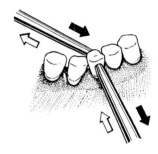

FIGURE 11-15. Determining the mobility of teeth with the handles of two dental instruments.

N (normal)	No movement noted clinically
1 degree	Movement of a tooth in both the facial and the lingual directions of up to and including 1 mm
2 degrees	Movement of a tooth in both the facial and lingual directions of greater than 1 mm
3 degrees	Movement of a tooth in both the facial and lingual directions of greater than 1 mm with easy depression

Tooth mobility is evaluated in a periodontal examination because it is one of the signs of periodontal tissue changes that can affect the outlook for successful treatment. In general, increased tooth mobility is related to one or more of the following pathological conditions:

1. Inflammation of the periodontium
2. Loss of periodontal support (bone loss)
3. Presence of occlusal trauma

The prognosis for successfully treating teeth with increased mobility varies, depending on the reasons for the mobility and the degree of control the therapist has over the causative factors. For example, if the teeth are loose because of inflammation related to plaque and calculus, the outlook for tightening the teeth is favorable following removal of the deposits and healing. However, if the mobility is primarily related to extensive loss of bone, the prognosis for tightening the teeth is less favorable.

The probing depth measurements and the mobility patterns should be recorded in the spaces provided on the dental chart (Fig. 11-5).

Radiographic analysis. The radiographic analysis of periodontal changes is helpful in assessing the extent of the periodontal tissue loss and in some instances noting etiological factors. However, radiographic findings should be verified with a clinical examination of the tissues involved. Periodontal disease cannot be diagnosed by viewing the radiographs alone because advanced periodontal soft tissue changes can occur and not be seen radiographically. However, an accurate radiographic survey used in conjunction with a clinical evaluation is an essential part of the periodontal examination.

Following are signs of periodontal changes that can be noted radiographically:

1. Integrity of the crestal lamina dura (Figs. 11-16 and 11-17, *B*). An indistinct representation of the crestal lamina dura suggests that bone has been destroyed but is not diagnostic.
2. Relationship of the crest of the interseptal bone to the adjacent cementoenamel junction (bone height or loss). The alveolar bone located on the facial and lingual root surfaces of the teeth cannot be seen radiographically.
3. Amount and general patterns of alveolar bone destruction—horizontal or angular (Fig. 11-17, *C* and *D*). Detailed osseous contours including the number of bony walls that form osseous defects, dehiscences, and fenestrations cannot be seen radiographically; however, the overall pattern of interproximal bone destruction can be noted.
4. Density of the supporting alveolar bone (Fig. 11-17, *E*).
5. Width of the periodontal ligament space on the mesial and distal surfaces of the teeth. However, the reliability of this finding is questionable because it varies considerably depending on the angle at which the radiograph is taken (Fig. 11-17, *F*).
6. Clinical-crown-to-clinical-root ratio (Fig. 11-17, *G*).
7. Large deposits of calculus and overhanging gingival margins of metallic restorations (Fig. 11-16, *I*).
8. Relation of periodontal destruction to anatomical structures (maxillary sinus).
9. Presence of periapical pathological changes.

Following are periodontal factors that *cannot* be determined through a radiographic evaluation alone:

1. Presence or absence of periodontal pockets
2. Success or failure of periodontal treatment
3. Topography (number of walls and contours) of osseous defects
4. Height or contour of bone located on the facial or lingual surfaces of the teeth
5. Presence or absence of occlusal trauma

Etiology of periodontal disease. Detecting the etiological factors for periodontal disease is an essential part of the examination because it not only aids in arriving at an accurate diagnosis and prognosis but it also outlines the conditions that must be corrected to eliminate the disease.

The periodontal examination should include a search for etiological factors in the following categories (mounted diagnostic models are a

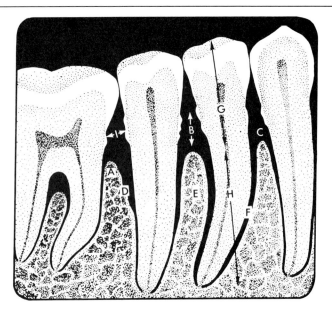

FIGURE 11-16. Radiographic changes consistent with periodontal disease. *A*, Indistinct crestal lamina dura. *B*, Increased distance between the crest of the interproximal alveolar bone and the cementoenamel junction. *C*, Horizontal pattern of alveolar bone resorption. *D*, Angular pattern of alveolar bone resorption. *E*, Decreased density of the supporting alveolar bone. *F*, Increased width of the periodontal ligament space. *G*, Increased length of the clinical crown caused by loss of supporting tissues. *H*, Decreased length of the clinical root related to the resorption of the periodontium. *I*, Calculus.

valuable aid in determining the predisposing and functional etiological factors):

1. Systemic (intrinsic) factors. Systemic factors can be evaluated through the medical history, physician consultation, physical evaluation, and laboratory examinations.
2. Local irritating (extrinsic) factors.
   a. Initiating factor is usually bacterial plaque, which is noted with disclosing solutions and a dental explorer. (Figs. 2-1 and 2-2, *A* and *B*).
   b. Predisposing factors such as calculus, overhanging gingival margins, open interproximal contact points (Figs. 2-4, 2-7, *A* and *B*), and malposed teeth are noted with the dental explorer, diagnostic casts, and intraoral radiographs. These findings should be noted on the dental chart.

3. Local functional factors, which include situations that can cause occlusal trauma. Examples are parafunctional habits (bruxism, clenching), occlusal prematurities, and severe loss of periodontal support. These factors are noted through the dental history, the functional analysis, the physical evaluation of the periodontium, and the radiographic analysis. A more detailed description of the examination for these factors is found in Chapter 8.

The etiology of many cases of periodontal disease is multifactorial and not always clear. However, noting the causative factors and categorizing them in such a way as to point out what role they are each playing in the patient's disease provide a basis for the determination of the prognosis and treatment plan. For more specific information concerning the etiology of

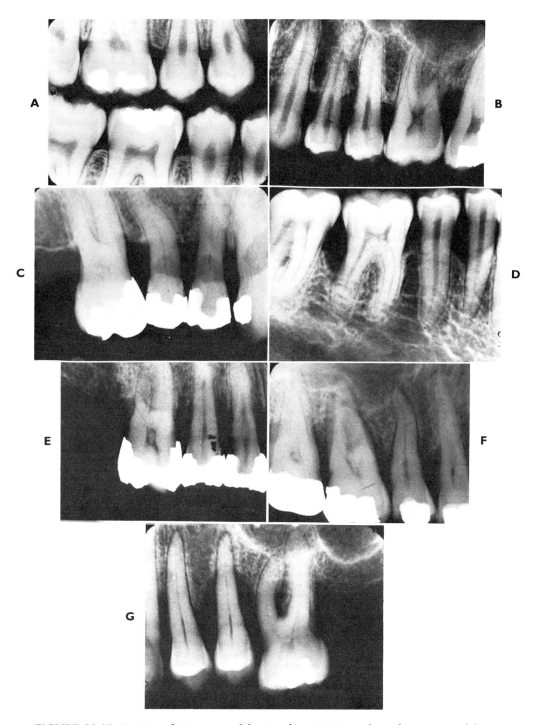

FIGURE 11-17. A, Note distinct crestal lamina dura. **B,** Note the indistinct crestal bone margin suggesting possible active bone resorption. **C,** Horizontal pattern of bone resorption. **D,** Angular pattern of bone resorption. **E,** Note the radiolucent areas in the coronal aspects of the interproximal alveolar bone. **F,** Note widened periodontal ligament spaces on the second premolar and first molar. These spaces are consistent with the lesion of occlusal trauma. **G,** Extensive bone loss on the second premolar suggests an unfavorable clinical-crown-to-clinical-root ratio.

periodontal disease consult Chapter 2 and each disease as it is discussed in other chapters.

PERIODONTAL DIAGNOSIS

Establishing the diagnosis of a specific periodontal case is a process in which the examiner uses all the information assembled about the patient to determine which of the recognized periodontal conditions best describes the disease present. The purpose of stating the diagnosis is to help the examiner determine the prognosis and treatment plan. This is made possible by the fact that most periodontal diagnostic terms denote the etiology as well as the nature of the disease process. Knowing the etiology is essential to determining the prognosis and treatment plan. An example of a proper diagnosis is "generalized gingivitis."

For more specific information about the diagnosis of specific disease entities, refer to the chapters in this book related to the conditions.

PERIODONTAL PROGNOSIS

The overall prognosis for a dentition affected by periodontal disease is the outlook for maintaining the dentition in periodontal health if comprehensive dental treatment is rendered. The individual prognosis should be established for certain teeth when conditions for them vary from those found throughout the mouth.

In general, the prognosis for retaining teeth in periodontal health that have been affected by periodontal disease is based on how much control the therapist and the patient have over the etiological factors. If the periodontal disease present can be related entirely to local etiological factors that are controllable, the prognosis is usually favorable. However, if the periodontal disease present is thought to be related, at least in part, to unknown or uncontrollable etiological agents, the prognosis is less favorable.

In the majority of patients the single most important factor in determining the prognosis is whether an adequate level of plaque control can be established over a long period of time.

In addition, the prognosis is based on which teeth remain with an adequate level of periodontal support. The support is necessary because periodontal health depends on adequate occlusal function as well as gingival health. Proper function cannot be reestablished unless an adequate number of teeth with the appropriate distribution and sufficient periodontal support remain to reestablish a physiological occlusion. More specific criteria for the prognosis of each individual periodontal condition are discussed in the chapters devoted to each disease.

PERIODONTAL TREATMENT PLAN

Determining the periodontal treatment plan consists of outlining all the procedures that must be performed to restore and maintain periodontal health and then integrating them into the total dental treatment plan. Periodontal treatment often involves restoration of lost tooth structure and correction of occlusal discrepancies as well as improving the plaque control, scaling, root planing, and pocket elimination procedures. Because of the interdependence of the procedures necessary to restore periodontal health, careful sequencing is essential if effective treatment is to be realized.

The periodontal portion of the dental treatment plan can be divided into the following three basic phases:

Phase I	Initial periodontal treatment
Phase II	Surgical access for thorough root planing, reduction of probing depths, correction of periodontal defects (pockets), and restoration of lost tooth structure and occlusal function.
Phase III	Periodontal maintenance

Phase I

Initial periodontal treatment is concerned with controlling as many of the etiological factors as possible without involving the patient in periodontal surgery or definitive restorative and prosthetic treatment. The following procedures are often included in initial treatment:

1. Treatment for any emergency situation

2. Medical treatment for established systemic etiological factors or conditions that would contraindicate or affect the results of the periodontal treatment
3. Instructions in personal oral hygiene (plaque control)
4. Scaling, root planing, and polishing of teeth
5. Removal of overhanging gingival margins of restorations
6. Treatment of deep carious lesions with temporary restorations
7. Endodontic therapy
8. Preliminary occlusal adjustment
9. Orthodontic treatment
10. Temporary crowns, bridges, and splints
11. Reevaluation of the periodontal health to include the effectiveness of the plaque control, the periodontal tissue response to the initial treatment, and the need for further treatment

At the termination of initial periodontal therapy for a patient with moderate to advanced periodontitis the plaque control should be effective, the gingival tissues should appear pink, firm, and noninflamed, but deep pockets which bleed upon probing will often persist. If so, surgical access for more definitive calculus removal, root planing, and possibly pocket reduction is usually indicated. This will provide a dentogingival environment more conducive to effective plaque control (Fig. 11-18). However, if adequate patient cooperation is not established during the initial therapy, periodontal surgery should be delayed until the patient's plaque control is adequate to prevent recurrence of the pockets following surgical treatment. If periodontal health is achieved during Phase I therapy, the patient is placed on a periodontal maintenance treatment program and Phase II is omitted (Fig. 11-19).

Phase II

Phase II involves establishing surgical access for more effective scaling and root planing, restoring lost tooth structure, and reestablishing a physiological occlusion. Following is a typical sequence of treatment for a patient who has moderate periodontitis with deep periodontal pockets (4 to 6 mm):

1. Periodontal surgery to improve the calculus removal and root preparation and to reduce periodontal pockets.
2. Postsurgical therapy until the periodontal tissues are healed
3. Occlusal adjustment
4. Reevaluation of the periodontal health
5. Definitive restorative and prosthetic treatment to include the following:
   a. Individual restorations to provide proper tooth contours and a physiologic occlusion
   b. Fixed and removable prosthetic appliances to replace missing teeth, to splint teeth together, and to restore a stable physiologic occlusion
6. Reevaluation of the periodontal tissues and, if healthy, a periodontal maintenance appointment in 3 months

Phase III

Periodontal maintenance treatment consists of a long-term sequence of treatment that is individually designed for each patient according to specific needs. The aim of this stage of treatment is to prevent the recurrence of the periodontal disease. The time interval between the periodontal maintenance appointments varies according to the effectiveness of the patient's plaque control, the rate of plaque and calculus formation, and the susceptibility to dental caries and periodontal disease. In general, this stage of treatment begins with 1- to 3-month intervals and is adjusted as the patient's needs are observed.

A typical periodontal maintenance appointment includes the following procedures:

1. Update of the patient's medical and dental history
2. Review of the patient's general health
3. Evaluation of the extraoral and intraoral soft tissues for any pathological changes
4. Reevaluation of the periodontal health to include an evaluation of the tissue ap-

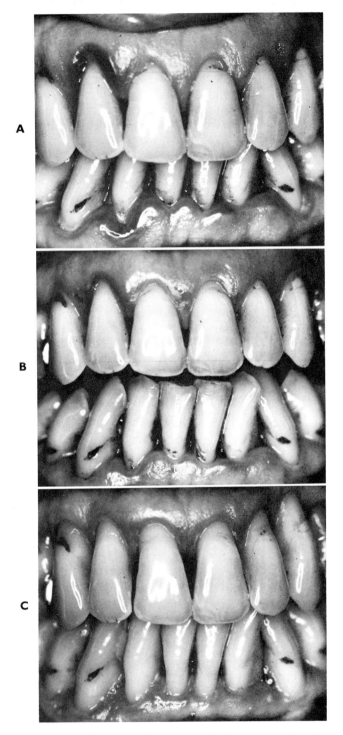

FIGURE 11-18. **A,** Generalized periodontitis and 5 to 7 mm periodontal pockets in 45-year-old woman. **B,** Same patient as **A** 1 month after instructions in plaque control and scaling and root planing of the teeth had been completed. The gingival inflammation has been reduced, but 4 to 6 mm pockets remain. **C,** Same patient 1 year after periodontal surgical procedures were done to reduce the pocket depths and create a dentogingival environment more conducive to effective plaque control.

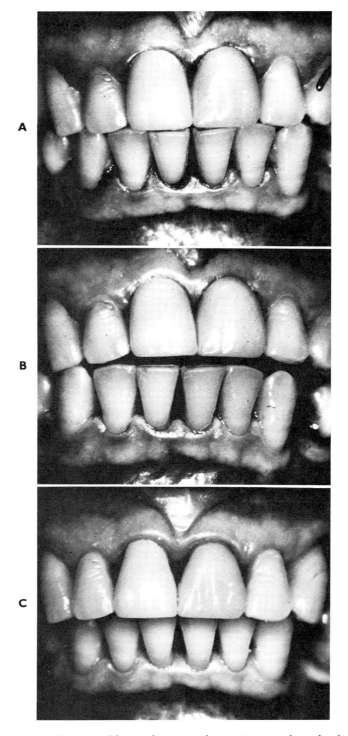

FIGURE 11-19. **A,** Chronic mild periodontitis with 3 to 5 mm probing depths in a 55-year-old woman. **B,** One month following instructions in plaque control and scaling and root planing. Note reduction in inflammation but persistent rounded contours and loosely adherent gingival tissues. **C,** The gingival tissues have undergone further healing 6 months following the procedures. The probing depths are 2 to 3 mm, and the tissues are more tapered and closely adherent to the teeth. No surgical treatment is indicated.

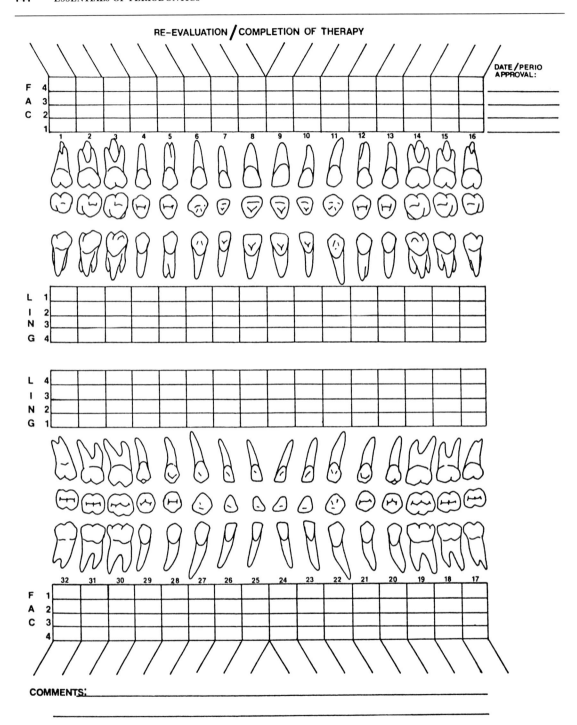

FIGURE 11-20. Dental chart designed for recording sequential probing depths at maintenance visits.

pearance and determination of probing depths and attachment levels (Fig. 11-20), tendency to bleed on instrumentation, and mobility patterns

5. Reevaluation of the occlusion, noting particularly the presence of wear facets, parafunctional habits, and occlusal prematurities
6. Reevaluation of the plaque control effectiveness by using disclosing solution and reviewing the patient's oral hygiene habits
7. Evaluation of the teeth for carious lesions by a clinical examination and periodic radiographic evaluation as needed
8. Thorough removal of all tooth deposits, smoothing of all root surfaces, and polishing of the teeth
9. Application of topical fluoride for patients who are particularly susceptible to dental caries and dental hypersensitivity
10. Discussion of the patient's progress, giving the patient the opportunity to ask periodontal health questions
11. Determination of the time interval before the next appointment

Effective long-term periodontal maintenance therapy is the most important of the three phases of treatment. Periodontal diseases are generally chronic in nature and tend to recur if the patient is not seen periodically for periodontal health reevaluation, encouragement and motivation for continued plaque control, and meticulous removal of all tooth deposits. Surgical periodontal treatment is of limited value without proper maintenance therapy.

SUGGESTED READINGS

American Dental Association: Accepted dental therapeutics, ed 37, Chicago, 1977, The Association, pp 3-18.

Carranza F: Glickman's clinical periodontology, ed 5, Philadelphia, 1979, WB Saunders Co, pp 549-605.

Hancock E, and Wirthlin M: The location of the periodontal probe tip in health and disease, J Periodontol 52:124, 1981.

Mahoney E, and Verdisco L: How to collect and record a health history, Philadelphia, 1976, JB Lippincott Co.

CHAPTER 12
Plaque Control in Periodontal Therapy

A significant relationship between the accumulation of bacterial plaque on the teeth and the development of gingivitis and periodontitis has been well established through clinical and epidemiological research. Loe, Theilade, and Jensen demonstrated in their experimental gingivitis study that stopping all efforts to control dental plaque in patients who have good periodontal health results in the development of gingivitis within 10 to 21 days and that reestablishing effective plaque control results in the elimination of the disease. In addition, a cross-sectional human study by Shei demonstrated an increase in alveolar bone resorption with poor oral hygiene. However, even though the cause-and-effect relationship between dental plaque and periodontal disease has been well established through clinical research, the biological mechanisms whereby the plaque microorganisms and their products initiate and maintain periodontal inflammation and tissue destruction are only beginning to be understood.

Effective plaque control is therefore the basis for the prevention and treatment of most inflammatory changes in the periodontal tissues. Plaque control refers to all the measures taken by both the patient and the dental team to prevent the accumulation of bacterial dental plaque and other deposits on the teeth and adjacent gingival surfaces. To date, plaque control is the most effective means of preventing the accumulation of microbial dental deposits and therefore preventing the initiation, devel-

opment, and progression of periodontal disease. The role of plaque control in the surgical management of periodontal disease has also been emphasized in recent investigations. Nyman, Lindhe, and Rosling have conducted human research studies which show that the effectiveness of the plaque control is directly related to the healing of periodontal surgical wounds. Their study demonstrated that when the patient's oral hygiene allowed continuous accumulation of bacterial plaque in the surgical areas, irrespective of the type of surgical procedure used, all procedures were equally ineffective in preventing the recurrence of periodontitis. In contrast, they found that 2 years following the performance of periodontal surgical procedures for patients who were placed on meticulous plaque control programs, similarly effective results occurred in terms of pocket elimination with a variety of surgical techniques. This finding is also consistent with the results of two long-term investigations conducted in private practice settings, which showed a strong positive relationship between periodontal therapy that included effective plaque control and the prolongation of natural dentitions.

The necessity for effective plaque control during the maintenance phase of treatment was pointed out by Chase when he stated that periodontal disease in the susceptible patient is not cured, only controlled. The continuous formation of dental plaque combined with the chronic nature of periodontal diseases means that long-term effective plaque control habits must be established to maintain periodontal health.

OBJECTIVES OF PLAQUE CONTROL

Regular effective plaque control has a twofold effect on the tissues. The primary role is the removal of soft deposits on the teeth and gingival tissues (dental plaque, materia alba, food debris). Gingival stimulation (gingival massage) may play a role in increasing gingival tone, surface keratinization, gingival vascularity, and gingival circulation; however, research findings in this area are not well established.

SEQUENCING OF ORAL HYGIENE INSTRUCTIONS IN THE PERIODONTAL TREATMENT PLAN

Patient instruction in plaque control and evaluation of the progress must be a continual process throughout the time the patient is undergoing treatment. However, time periods exist within the treatment plan when specific goals must be accomplished.

Initial therapy

The first form of active periodontal therapy should usually be instructions in oral hygiene. If this is begun before the removal of calculus, the patients receive the benefit of experiencing a reduction in the tendency for gingival bleeding through their own efforts alone (Fig. 12-1, A and B). This method is an effective way to have the patients learn how important their cotherapist efforts are in the periodontal treatment.

If the deposits of calculus or the nature of the restorative dentistry are such that they prevent the removal of plaque through normal patient oral hygiene methods, initial professional debridement is performed before giving the instructions in plaque control (Fig. 12-2). A maximal level of plaque control may not be possible during the initial therapy because of the presence of pockets; however, surgical peri-odontal treatment should not be initiated unless the patient is practicing a level of plaque control that is adequate to maintain periodontal health following pocket reduction procedures.

Surgical therapy

Oral hygiene reinforcement and the introduction of modified techniques following the periodontal surgical procedures should be started during the postoperative visit in which the periodontal dressing is removed and continued during subsequent appointments (Fig. 12-3, A to C). Maximal pocket reduction and minimal tooth sensitivity following periodontal surgery are directly related to the effectiveness of the plaque control during the initial healing phases.

Restorative and prosthetic treatment

Proper instructions on how to clean fixed prosthodontic restorations, fixed splints, and removable appliances are as important as their construction and should be considered an integral part of the prosthetic service.

Periodontal maintenance therapy

Even though a high level of plaque control is achieved during the active phases of treatment, periodic professional review of the patient's progress and techniques is essential for long-term effectiveness. In view of the chronic nature of periodontal disease, this review is the most important phase of periodontal treatment. The prevention of root caries and tooth hypersensitivity also depends on the long-term continuation of effective plaque control.

ORAL HYGIENE AIDS
Antimicrobial control of dental plaque

Mechanical methods are the principal means of preventing the accumulation and succession of bacterial plaque and other tooth deposits. However, research has shown that various chemical antimicrobial agents, when used in conjunction with conventional therapeutic methods, can be helpful in the control of su-

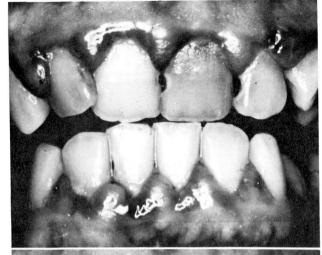

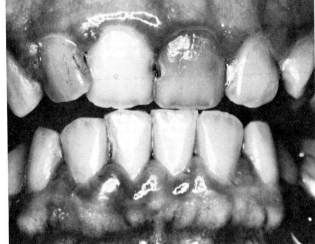

FIGURE 12-1. **A,** Adult patient with generalized periodontitis. **B,** Same patient 1 week following instructions in oral hygiene. Note the reduction in inflammation.

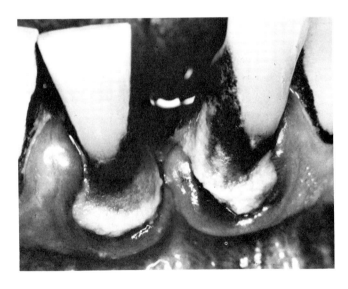

FIGURE 12-2. Heavy calculus, which must be removed before instructions in oral hygiene to allow access to the gingival sulcus for plaque removal.

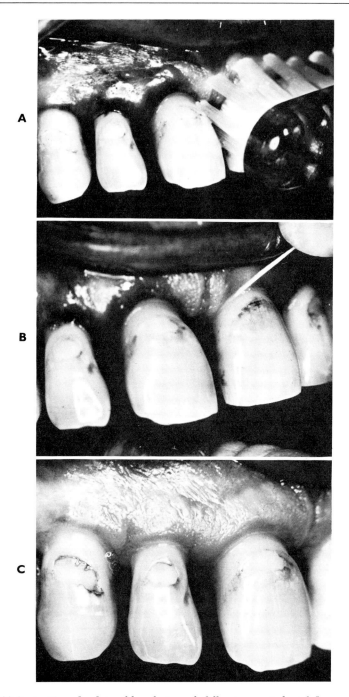

FIGURE 12-3. A, Use of soft toothbrush 1 week following periodontal flap surgery. **B,** Use of dental floss 1 week following periodontal flap surgery. **C,** Healed gingival tissues 2 months following periodontal surgery and effective plaque control.

pragingival plaque and gingivitis. Antimicrobial agents can also be applied subgingivally by irrigating devices, but currently the subgingival penetration and effectiveness is minimal. Antibiotics have been effectively applied subgingivally through slow-release devices, but the methods are not in general use at this time. For chemical antiplaque agents to be useful in the treatment of established periodontitis they must be able to affect the subgingival plaque.

Antimicrobial agents can be administered systemically or applied topically. Antibiotics such as penicillin, tetracycline, and metronidazole are generally administered systemically while antiseptic agents such as chlorhexidine, phenolic compounds, fluorides, and sanguinarine are incorporated into mouthrinses and/or dentifrices.

In evaluating products for use it is important to consider their effectiveness and safety. Of particular concern in these agents is their ability to not only alter or decrease plaque formation but to also prevent or decrease periodontal diseases. In 1986 the Council on Dental Therapeutics of the American Dental Association (CDT-ADA) issued the following guidelines for the evaluation of chemotherapeutic products for the control of supragingival plaque and gingivitis;*

1. Characteristics of the study population should be representative of typical product users.
2. Active product should be used in normal regimen and compared with a placebo control, or, where applicable, an active control.
3. Crossover or parallel designed studies are acceptable.
4. Studies should be a minimum of 6 months in duration.
5. Two studies conducted by independent investigators are required.
6. Microbiological sampling should estimate

plaque qualitatively to complement indexes that measure plaque quantitatively.
7. Plaque and gingivitis scoring and microbiological sampling should be conducted at baselines, 6 months, and an intermediate period.
8. Microbiological profile should demonstrate that pathogenic or opportunistic microorganisms do not develop over the course of the study.
9. The toxicological profile of products should include carcinogenicity and mutagenicity assays in addition to generally recognized tests for drug safety.

When considering the recommendation or use of various products for patients, it is important to know whether the manufacturer of the drug followed these guidelines in evaluating the product. At this time the mouthrinses meeting these standards are a chlorhexidine product, Peridex, which is available by prescription only, and a product containing phenol, Listerine, which is available over the counter.

Antibiotics

The principle antibiotic drugs used in periodontal therapy are tetracycline, metronidazole, and penicillin, but other agents have also been shown to depress oral microorganisms when administered systemically.

Tetracycline administered systemically are concentrated and excreted in the gingival sulcus with the sulcular fluid. It is particularly effective against the microorganism *Actinobacillus actinomycetemcomitans* and has been shown to be beneficial in the treatment of juvenile periodontitis when used in conjunction with local debridement and surgery. It has also been suggested for treatment of "refractory" periodontitis but has not been shown to have long-range advantages in the treatment of adult periodontitis. While the serious side effects are minimal, tetracycline should not be used for patients with a history of liver damage. It is

---

*Council on Dental Therapeutics of the American Dental Association, JADA 112-529, 1986.

also now recognized that the effectiveness of birth control pills can be significantly reduced by tetracycline. Local delivery of tetracycline in hollow fibers is an effective way to deliver the drug subgingivally. The fibers are placed into the pocket for 10 days and then removed. Substantial changes in the subgingival microflora have been shown.

Metronidazole is effective against gram-negative anaerobes and spirochetes and has been utilized in the treatment of various periodontal diseases, including acute necrotizing ulcerative gingivitis and periodontitis. It should not be administered in conjunction with the use of alcohol.

Penicillin has been shown to suppress plaque formation. It may be used in the treatment of acute periodontal conditions and in conjunction with certain periodontal surgical procedures. It is the drug of choice for the treatment of many serious diseases. Because of the tendency to develop resistant strains of bacteria during its use, it is not justified in the treatment of most periodontal diseases.

Oral antimicrobial agents

Many agents have been studied for their effectiveness in treating oral conditions. In addition to a proven effectiveness against periodontal diseases, the following characteristics are considered important for antimicrobial agents: lack of toxicity, poor absorption from the gastrointestinal system, broad rather than specific antibacterial spectrum, low drug-resistance development, and substantivity. Substantivity, as used in this context, refers to the abilities of a drug to be absorbed to a surface and then released at therapeutically effective levels.

Kornman has suggested that topically applied antimicrobial agents be classified according to their substantivity. First generation agents kill oral bacteria but do not have substantivity and are therefore less effective. Second generation agents have substantivity and not only kill oral bacteria but adhere to the teeth and are more effective in controlling the

growth of bacterial plaque. In recent years there has been particular interest in the following products: chlorhexidine, oxygenating agents, phenolic compounds, quaternary ammonium agents, stannous fluoride, and sanguinarine.

Chlorhexidine digluconate is the most effective topical antimicrobial agent in reducing plaque and gingivitis, with short- and long-term studies reporting 45% average reduction in gingivitis and 55% average reduction in plaque. The mode of action is reduction in pellicle formation, alteration of the bacteria's ability to attach to teeth, and disruption of the bacterial cell wall. Chlorhexidine digluconate has high substantivity which includes the ability not only to adhere to the oral structures but also to be released slowly. It is available in the United States in a 0.12% concentration as the prescription mouthrinse Peridex. The recommended dosage is to rinse with one half an ounce of the drug twice a day after meals and after the use of other oral hygiene aids. The side effects are staining of the teeth, alteration of taste, increase in calculus formation, and reversible desquamation of oral epithelium in young children. Long-term studies did not show the development of resistant bacterial strains. The drug is recommended as an adjunct to mechanical plaque control therapy in the prevention and treatment of gingivitis. It is also helpful immediately following periodontal surgery.

Oxygenating agents have been used orally for many years, and their antiinflammatory properties may be helpful in suppressing the symptoms of certain oral conditions. However, long-term studies of the effect of oxygenating agents in the treatment of periodontal diseases are not available, and short-term findings are not consistent. Oral ulcerations have been noted with the use of hydrogen peroxide.

Phenolic compounds have been studied in both the short and long terms, with 25% to 30% reductions in plaque and gingivitis noted. Listerine, the most common product in this category, consists of three phenol-derived essential oils: thymol, menthol, and eucalyptol combined with methylsalicylate. It is delivered in a vehicle of 26.9% alcohol and has a pH of 5.0. This product also alters the bacterial cell wall. It has low substantivity but a high safety factor.

Quaternary ammonium compounds have been shown to reduce plaque but have varied effects on gingival health. Cetylpyridinium chloride is a common agent in this category and is found in Cepacol and Scope. These agents work by increasing the permeability of the bacterial cell wall, which decreases the bacterial metabolism, increases the cell lysis, and reduces the bacteria's ability to attach to tooth surfaces. They have low substantivity but are very safe.

Stannous fluorides have been shown to suppress plaque formation, but long-term studies on their effect on plaque and gingival index scores have been disappointing. The product is most often supplied as an agueous gel, a 0.3% to 0.4% concentration being the most effective. The antibacterial activity may be related to the tin ion. It has moderate substantivity and a limited shelf life.

Sanguinarine is a chemical derived from the bloodroot plant (Sanguinaria canadensis). The product includes sanguinarine and zinc chloride in an alcohol vehicle. It is available in a mouthrinse and a dentifrice. It has low substantivity and a pH of 3.0 in the mouthrinse and 4.0 in the dentifrice. It acts by altering the bacterial cell surface to reduce its ability to aggregate and attach. The short-term studies on the use of both the mouthrinse and the dentifrice four times each day showed some plaque and gingivitis reduction, but the long-term study did not show the same effectiveness.

Toothbrushing

The toothbrush is the fundamental tool for the mechanical removal of plaque and other deposits.

Toothbrushes come in a variety of sizes, shapes, bristle textures, length, and bristle arrangement to meet the patient's individual needs. No one toothbrush has been shown to be superior. The American Dental Association has not evaluated each brush as to its particular merit but has established certain guidelines regarding acceptability. According to the American Dental Association, toothbrushes should have a brushing surface from 1 to 1¼ inches long and 5/16 to 3/8 inch wide, two to four rows, five to 12 tufts per row. The following points should also be taken into consideration when selecting and recommending a toothbrush:

1. Type of toothbrush selected for a patient depends on the needs of the individual rather than the superiority of any particular type of brush. No one toothbrush is adequate for all patients.
2. Proper brush should provide easy accessibility to all areas of the mouth. Small-headed brushes are often helpful in this regard.
3. Brush should clean efficiently and be easy for the patient to manipulate.
4. Nylon bristles are recommended.
5. Brush should be compatible with the recommended brushing technique.
6. Two brushes are recommended to be used alternately. They should be replaced when the bristles start bending or fraying.

Mechanical or motor-driven toothbrushes

Many types of power-driven toothbrushes are on the market today. These brushes employ several different types of stroke action. Numerous research studies have been conducted regarding the superiority of power-driven versus manual toothbrushes. Controversy does exist over the superiority of the electric versus the manual brush. The majority of the long-term studies have not indicated the automatic brush to be more effective than the manual in removing plaque. Patients who are adequately instructed can remove plaque as well with a hand brush as with an automatic brush. One exception is the superior subgingival and interproximal cleansing of the Interplak Home Plaque Removal Instrument. Automatic brushes do have certain advantages for handicapped individuals, hygienically lazy children and adults, and patients with orthodontic appliances. They are also helpful if one has to brush another person's teeth.

Toothbrushing methods

No one method of toothbrushing is adequate to meet the needs of all patients. The thoroughness of the removal of deposits is more important than the technique in evaluating the effectiveness of toothbrushing. Several specific techniques of brushing have been developed, and the selection of a method depends on the individual situation.

Following is a list of certain criteria that should be assessed when selecting a toothbrush and a toothbrushing technique for the individual patient. These suggestions are based on the fact that the brush and the technique selection are not arbitrary decisions but based on certain indications and contraindications. It is important for the patient to realize that toothbrushing cleans the facial and lingual surfaces of the teeth primarily and that interproximal oral hygiene aids must be used to clean the interproximal tooth surfaces.

I. Patient's clinical situation
  A. State of gingival and periodontal tissues in regard to health or disease (examples of the tissues' clinical characteristics that influence the method of choice in toothbrushing)
    1. Tissue state (contour, tone, texture, size)—normal, fibrotic, bulbous, edematous, enlarged
    2. Papillary contour—open or filled embrasure spaces
    3. Pocket or sulcular depth
  B. Anatomical limitations
    1. Size and contour of the dental arch
    2. Position, inclination, and contour of the individual teeth
    3. Presence of edentulous areas and replacement for the missing teeth

II. Patient's personal situation
  A. Patient's level of manual dexterity
  B. Motivational level, ability, and willingness of the patient to act on recommended procedures

Brushing sequence and timing. Regardless of the toothbrushing method selected, a sequence of brushing should be given to the patient. This pattern in brushing is important to ensure that the patient brushes all areas consistently. It is recommended that the patient be instructed to start with the molar region of one arch around the opposite side, then continue back around the lingual or facial surfaces of the same arch. The same procedure is then followed on the other arch until all accessible surfaces are cleaned. The last surfaces to be brushed are the occlusals. The number of strokes applied to each area or time spent cleaning an area is equally important as establishing a systematic routine. Depending on the particular needs of the patient and the method of brushing used, the patient is instructed to stroke each area ten times or spend 10 seconds per area, then move on to the next area.

Several toothbrushing methods are commonly in use.

Bass method (intrasulcular method). If the Bass method is properly performed, it is efficient at removing dental plaque from the gingival third of the tooth (gingival margin) and from shallow gingival sulci. This method is designed to direct soft bristles of 0.007-inch uniform thickness with rounded filament ends into the gingival sulcus (Fig. 12-4). A vibratory motion is then used to break up the subgingival plaque colonies as well as those in the gingival third of the tooth.

On the facial surfaces of all teeth and on the lingual surfaces of the posterior teeth the head of the brush is placed parallel with the occlusal surfaces of the teeth and the bristles are directed apically into the gingival sulcus at a 45-degree angle to the long axes of the teeth. The toothbrush is activated by applying gentle pres-

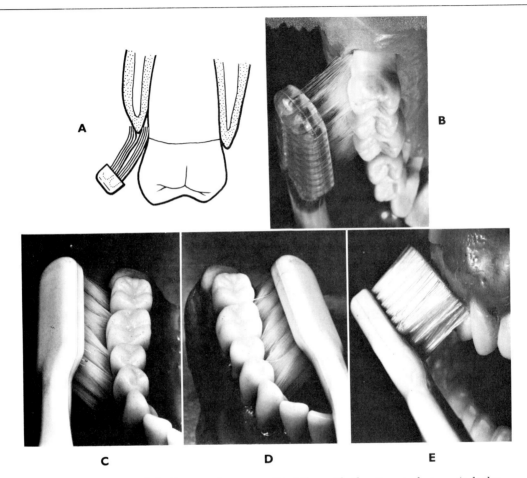

FIGURE 12-4. A and **B.** Proper placement of bristles with the Bass technique (sulcular brushing). Notice how the ends of the bristles are inserted into the gingival sulcus. The brush is activated with a slight vibratory motion. **C,** Brush placement on the buccal surfaces of the mandibular posterior teeth. **D,** Brush placement on the lingual surfaces of the mandibular posterior teeth. **E,** Brush placement on the buccal surfaces of the maxillary posterior teeth.

sure in an apical direction and by making short vibratory strokes. The ends of the bristles should not move from tooth to tooth, and vigorous forces are not necessary. Accurate brush placement and the use of gentle pressure should be emphasized to prevent gingival abrasions caused by haphazard horizontal scrubbing strokes commonly used.

On the lingual surfaces of the anterior teeth it is recommended that the brush be placed in a vertical direction parallel with the long axes of the teeth and only one or two teeth be brushed at a time. Apical pressure with a vibratory motion is used in these areas as well.

Modified Bass method. The first part of the modified Bass method is identical to the Bass technique. The modification consists of sweeping the bristles downward over the tooth surface occlusally after completing the vibratory motion in the gingival sulcus.

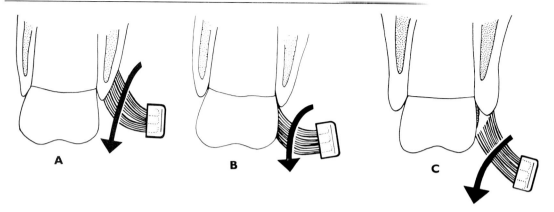

FIGURE 12-5. Roll technique. The bristles are first directed apically as in **A** and then swept in an occlusal direction with a rolling motion as in **B. C,** Rolled gingival margin prevents removal of plaque from sulcular area.

Roll method (Fig. 12-5, *A* to *C*). The roll method is popular because it requires less skill to perform and less time to teach than the other techniques. With ideal tapering gingival contours, this method is effective. However, when rolled gingival margins or prominent contours of the attached gingiva are present, the risk exists that the ends of the bristles will move from the crest of the gingiva to the tooth surfaces without reaching the vulnerable sulcular area (Fig. 12-5, *C*). Most toothbrushes are suitable for this method, although a softer multitufted nylon brush may be the most effective. With this technique the sides of the bristles are placed on the attached gingiva with the bristles directed apically and the jaws separated; then the sides of the bristles are pressed against the gingiva to produce a blanching effect. With continued pressure the brush is slowly rolled down over the gingiva and tooth surface by rotating the wrist. This stroke is repeated at least five times for each area before the next area is cleaned. It is important to overlap brush placement when moving to the adjacent position to ensure no area is missed.

Stillman's method. With Stillman's technique the bristle ends are placed at a 45-degree angle with the bristles directed apically on the gingiva and partly on the cervical por-

tion of the teeth. Once the bristles are in place pressure is applied to blanch the gingiva and a gentle but firm vibratory-rotary motion is applied to the brush with the bristles remaining in the same position (Fig. 12-6, *A*).

Modified Stillman's technique. The only difference between Stillman's and modified Stillman's technique is that with modified Stillman's technique a rolling stroke is used after the vibratory motion (Fig. 12-6, *B*). The Stillman and modified Stillman methods provide stimulation to the gingival tissues and remove soft deposits from the cervical areas of the tooth surface.

Charter's method. The Charter method may be used when the interdental gingiva does not fill the embrasure spaces. With open interproximal embrasure spaces this technique provides a greater potential for cleaning the mesial and distal surfaces of teeth. Research has indicated that neither the roll nor Bass methods are effective in cleaning interproximal tooth surfaces. This technique is contraindicated when full interdental embrasure spaces exist. With this method the bristles are placed at a 45-degree angle directed toward the occlusal surface. The sides of the bristles are then placed against the marginal gingiva and the tooth, extending the bristles into the interproximal spaces. A firm

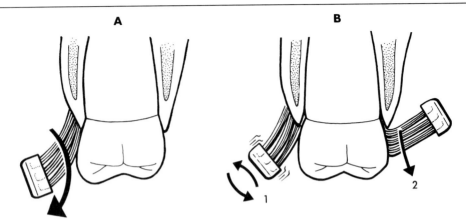

FIGURE 12-6. A, Stillman's technique. The bristles are directed apically and compressed laterally against the gingiva. A vibratory rotary motion is used to activate the brush. **B,** Modified Stillman's technique. Following the vibratory motion shown at *1*, the brush is moved occlusally with a rolling motion over the gingiva and tooth surface, as shown in *2*.

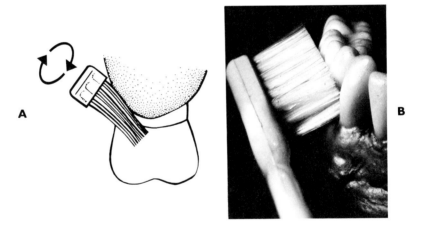

FIGURE 12-7. A and **B,** Charter's technique. The bristles are directed occlusally, and the sides of the bristles are firmly flexed against the gingiva with a vibratory motion.

rotary-vibratory movement is used while keeping the bristles in position. (Fig. 12-7). This technique is difficult to learn and is not as frequently recommended as it has been in the past.

Brushing the occlusal surfaces

A common error in brushing the occlusal surfaces is the use of long scrubbing strokes over all the occlusal surfaces. To properly clean these surfaces the brush bristles are placed at a right angle on the occlusal surfaces with the ends of the bristles deep into the pits and fissures. Two types of strokes are recommended. Using a circular motion, vibrate the brush while keeping the bristles in position. Force the bristles into the pits and fissures and, using sharp, quick strokes, lift the brush to remove deposits. After one area is completed, the brush is then moved to the next area, overlapping the area previously brushed.

Brushing the tongue

It has been suggested that patients brush not only the teeth but also the tongue. Microorganisms, soft debris, and desquamated epithelial cells should be removed from the dorsum of the tongue. This is done by placing the bristles at a right angle on the tongue with the bristles directed toward the throat. Apply pressure as the brush is brought forward across the surface of the tongue.

Mouth rinsing

After brushing or using any other cleaning aid, mouth rinsing is important to flush away the debris that was loosened but not removed. Water or a mouthwash should be swished vigorously throughout the mouth.

Toothbrush trauma

Toothbrush trauma refers to any negative side effects (injury) that result from improper use of the toothbrush. This injury can affect the soft tissues and/or the tooth itself. Following are the most common causes of toothbrush trauma:

1. Excessive pressure
2. Incorrect brush angulation
3. Bristle consistency too hard
4. Incorrect brush direction (horizontal brushing)
5. Puncture of the gingiva with the bristles
6. Use of a toothbrush with frayed bristles

Adjuncts to toothbrushing

Toothbrushing alone cannot completely clean all the surfaces of the teeth. For ideal plaque control toothbrushing should be supplemented with aids that assist in cleaning the interproximal as well as other protected tooth surfaces that are missed by a toothbrush. Devices are also available that are used primarily to massage the gingiva. These aids are meant to supplement toothbrushing, and by no means are

they intended to replace or substitute for the toothbrush. The various supplemental aids given to a patient to obtain or maintain optimal oral health will depend on the individual's clinical condition.

Interproximal cleaning aids

The need for regular removal of plaque from the interproximal tooth surface is emphasized by the fact that the most frequent site of periodontal disease is in the interdental periodontal tissues. Toothbrushing is not usually effective for the removal of interproximal plaque and debris. Because of this fact, various aids have been developed for cleaning interproximal areas. The use and selection of these aids depend on the clinical characteristics of the embrasure spaces, the condition of the gingival tissues, and the patient's individual needs regarding rate and location of dental plaque accumulation.

Dental floss. For patients who have healthy periodontal tissues and have not experienced interproximal periodontal recession, dental floss provides maximal access and cleaning effectiveness for flat or convex proximal tooth surfaces (Figs. 12-8 and 12-9, *A*). The use of dental floss is also recommended for patients who have lost interdental tissues, but it should be remembered that it is less effective on concave root surfaces (Fig. 12-9, *B*).

Several types of dental floss or dental type are available. Unwaxed dental floss has been suggested to be more effective in plaque removal than waxed floss; however, research has not supported this concept. Clinically patients with rough restorations or extremely tight interproximal contact points find waxed floss easier to use because it does not shred or break as quickly. Tufted floss is also available.

Several different ways to use floss exist. Whichever method is employed, the following principles should be kept in mind for optimal use:

1. Floss should be securely anchored around one finger of each hand and then

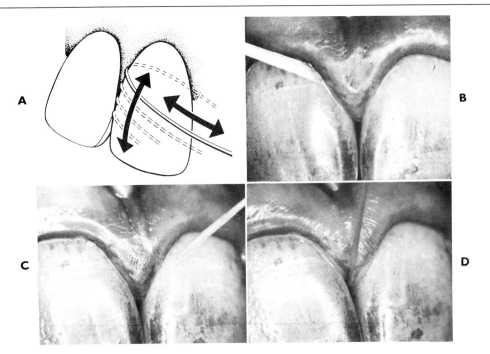

FIGURE 12-8. Dental floss use. **A,** Note that the floss is wrapped around the facial and lingual embrasures to facilitate maximal plaque removal. **B,** Use of floss on the mesial surface of the maxillary right central incisor. **C,** Use of floss on the mesial surface of the adjacent right central incisor. **D,** Avoid traumatizing the interdental gingiva.

a small length (1 to 2 inches) should be stretched between the guiding fingers (Fig. 12-10).

2. Clean floss should be used in each area.
3. Floss should not be forced or snapped past the contact point into the sulcus or gingiva because this practice can injure the soft tissue. The floss should be gently worked through the interproximal contact points.
4. Floss should first be placed at the base of the gingival sulcus, and it should be moved in an up-and-down motion between the sulcus and the interproximal contact point.
5. Floss is moved along the tooth surface, not the gingival surface. The floss is curved around the tooth, not just straight in (Fig. 12-8). Care should be taken to avoid cutting the gingival tissues.

6. Flossing should be done slowly to avoid sloppy, incorrect technique and trauma (Fig. 12-8, *D*).
7. If the patient lacks the dexterity to use the floss properly, one of the several commercial floss holders available should be recommended (Fig. 12-11).
8. Several types of bridge threaders are available for flossing under fixed bridges (Fig. 12-12, *A* and *B*).
9. Patient's flossing techniques should be checked regularly to ensure correct and effective usage.

Balsa wood wedge toothpick. The wedge toothpick (Stim-u-Dent) is made of a soft wood and is triangular in shape to contour to the interdental spaces. It is contraindicated for areas where the interdental gingiva fills the interdental embrasure spaces. If used when the embrasure spaces are full, it creates a space and can

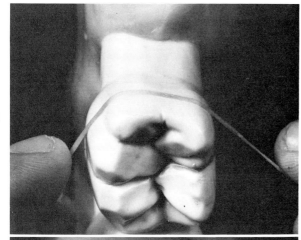

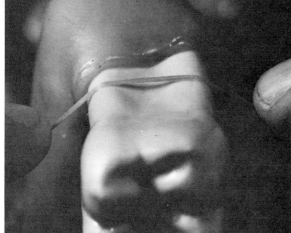

FIGURE 12-9. A, Effective use of dental tape on convex teeth surfaces. **B,** Ineffective use of dental tape on concave interproximal tooth surfaces.

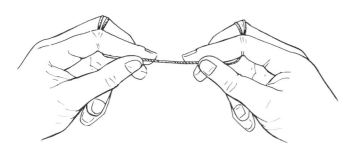

FIGURE 12-10. Effective method of holding dental floss. Note that only a small length of floss should be left between the principal guiding fingers.

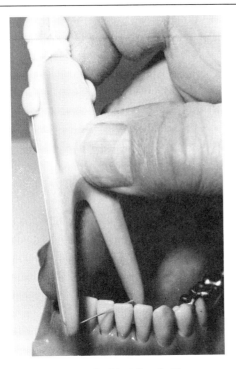

FIGURE 12-11. Floss holder.

injure the tissue. If used properly as a supplement to brushing, it is effective in removing plaque and debris, stimulating the gingiva, and recontouring the interdental gingiva.

The toothpick is first moistened in the mouth to soften it. It is then placed interproximally with the base of the triangle toward the gingiva and at a slight angle toward the crown (Fig. 12-13). The toothpick is pressed firmly against the proximal surfaces of the adjacent teeth. The toothpick is then moved in and out or up and down, depending on the size of the interdental space. This procedure is repeated several times in each area. One limitation of the Stim-U-Dent is that it is hard to insert from the lingual aspects. The patient should be instructed that these are special toothpicks and not to substitute regular wooden toothpicks (except the Perio-Aid toothpick) because any other type can cause tissue trauma. Plastic tips (P/S, Polisher-Stimulator) are also available.

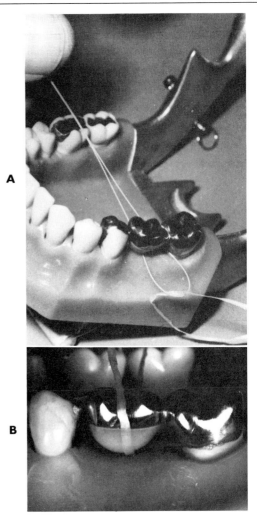

FIGURE 12-12. A, Plastic leader to help thread floss under fixed bridges and between splinted teeth. **B,** Cleaning the gingival surface of a pontic with dental tape.

They resemble the balsa wood wedges in appearance and technique of use.

Toothpicks in special holders. Small round polished toothpicks can be placed in special plastic handles. The Perio-Aid is an example. This handle allows more flexibility in placing the toothpick from the lingual aspects and in other areas with limited access. The Perio-Aid also enables the patient to reach into exposed

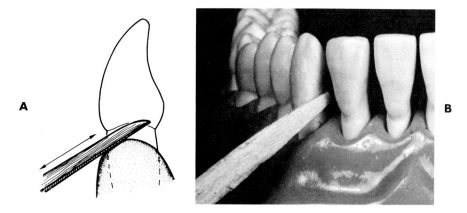

FIGURE 12-13. A and **B,** Proper placement of the balsa wood wedge toothpick against the proximal surface of a tooth. It is activated with an in-and-out motion, pressing firmly against the tooth surface.

furcations and other concave surfaces of teeth (Fig. 12-14).

Interdental brushes. Small cone-shaped or tapered brushes are particularly helpful in cleaning large open interdental embrasure spaces and furcations. These brushes can adapt easily to irregular and concave tooth surfaces. They should be inserted into the interdental space and moved back and forth in a faciolingual direction. If the brush is slightly larger than the embrasure space, it is more effective (Fig. 12-15, *A* to *C*).

Gauze strips, pipe cleaners, and yarn. Gauze strips, pipe cleaners, and yarn are effective cleaning aids in special situations. Pipe cleaners are effective for cleaning open furcation areas. The pipe cleaner is passed through the furcation with a back-and-forth movement. Gauze strips and four-ply cotton yarn are effective aids for cleaning the proximal surfaces of teeth adjacent to edentulous areas and open embrasure spaces. The gauze strips and yarn are placed on the proximal surfaces of the teeth and moved back and forth in a "shoeshine motion." In pipe cleaners and cotton yarn white is recommended to avoid dyes.

Rubber tip interdental stimulators—gingival massage or stimulation. Controversy exists over the importance and significance of gingival massage and its role in gingival health. It has been reported that gingival massage produces epithelial thickening, increased keratinization, and increased mitotic activity in the oral epithelium and connective tissues of the gingiva. It is also claimed that circulation of the gingiva is improved. Clinical observations indicate that interdental gingival massage may aid in reshaping bulbous gingiva and stimulate healing following periodontal surgery. While gingival massage may seem to have some clinical value in maintaining periodontal health, no controlled research exists to support this view. The emphasis in oral hygiene should be placed on plaque control rather than gingival massage.

The rubber tip stimulator is conical in shape and is available at the end of the handle of some toothbrushes or attached to a separate handle. The rubber tip stimulator is contraindicated when the embrasure spaces are full. In this situation they should only be used along the gingival sulcus on the proximal surfaces. With open embrasures the rubber tip is inserted interproximally at a 45-degree angle with the tip pointed in an occlusal direction. The stimulator is activated by applying pressure with a vibratory or rotary motion (Fig. 12-16). This procedure is done on both the facial and the lingual sides.

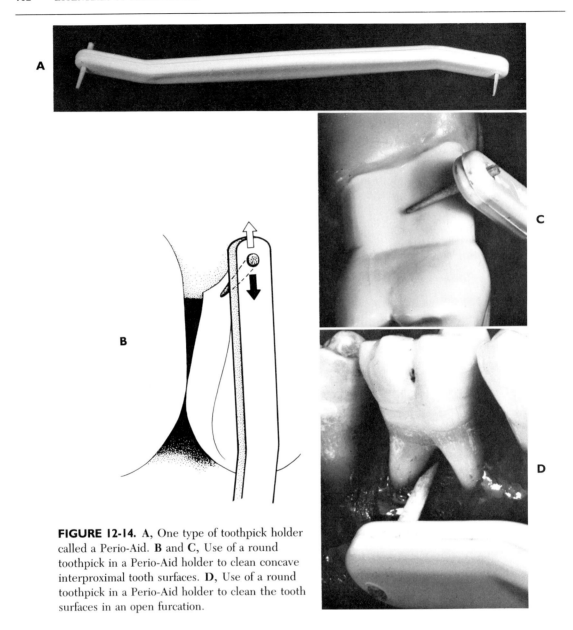

FIGURE 12-14. A, One type of toothpick holder called a Perio-Aid. **B** and **C,** Use of a round toothpick in a Perio-Aid holder to clean concave interproximal tooth surfaces. **D,** Use of a round toothpick in a Perio-Aid holder to clean the tooth surfaces in an open furcation.

Disclosing tablets and solutions

The ability to see what is to be removed from the teeth is helpful to the patient. While large amounts of dental plaque can be seen or felt in the mouth by the experienced patient, plaque is generally invisible and must be stained for patient observation. In addition, the disclosing of plaque helps the patient learn the difference between bacterial dental plaque and food debris. A patient generally knows that it is desirable to remove food debris, which is relatively easily seen or felt, but the need to remove the more tenaciously attached colorless plaque is not always recognized. These stains aid in patient

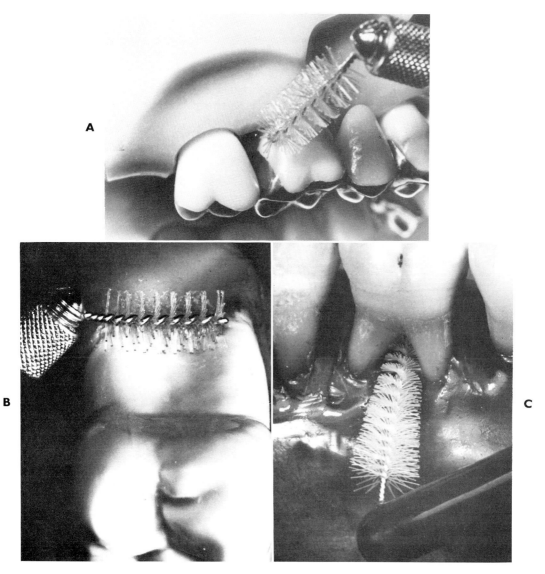

FIGURE 12-15. A, Use of a small brush in a handle to clean the tooth surfaces in an open embrasure space. **B,** Use of an interproximal brush to clean a concave tooth surface. **C,** Use of an interproximal brush to clean an open furcation.

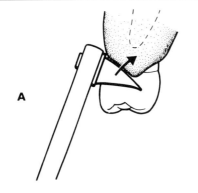

FIGURE 12-16. A, Rubber stimulator is placed firmly against the interdental gingiva at a 45-degree angle to the tooth. It is activated with a vibratory motion directed against the gingiva. **B,** Use of rubber stimulator in the maxillary anterior region. **C,** Use of the rubber stimulator in an open furcation area.

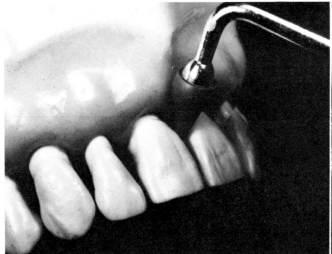

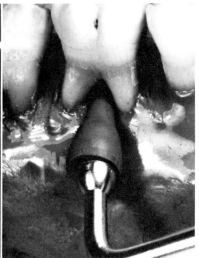

education, motivation, and home care because the patient can use these dyes to judge the effectiveness of the oral hygiene routine. Various studies have shown that the use of plaque-disclosing dyes can improve the effectiveness of oral hygiene instructions. We recommend that they be used to show the patient where the plaque accumulates on the teeth and what oral hygiene techniques are needed to remove it. The patient uses the disclosing wafers at home to monitor personal progress. Daily use is recommended at first, and then periodically after the plaque removal techniques have been perfected. Minimal plaque scores can be used to stimulate the patient to achieve more effective plaque control.

The disclosing stains come in tablet and liquid form. They are water soluble and stain plaque blue, purple, or red, depending on the type of stain used. These stains are contraindicated for patients who have a large number of synthetic restorations. Examples of disclosing solutions are Bismark Brown solution, erythrosine (FDC Red number 3), and sodium fluorescein dye.

Dentifrices

A dentifrice contains abrasives, detergents, and flavoring agents. The detergents and abrasives aid in polishing and help in the removal of the debris. The flavoring agents give a pleasant taste to brushing. While chemically active antiplaque agents, stannous fluoride, and sanguinarine are available in commercial dentifrices, their effect is minimal, and the plaque and debris are principally dislodged and removed by the mechanical action of the toothbrush rather than the chemical action of the dentifrice. In recent years a mixture of bicarbonate of soda and hydrogen peroxide has been suggested as an aid in cleaning the mouth. While extensive claims have been made in support of this material, controlled studies have shown no differences in gingival inflammation between patients using bicarbonate-peroxide and patients using regular toothpaste as long as deep scaling of the teeth was performed first. Some dentifrices now contain soluble pyrophosphates, which are crystal-growth inhibitors that interrupt the transformation of amorphous calcium phosphate into dental calculus. When used as an adjunct to regular professional care and personal oral hygiene procedures, dentifrices containing these compounds have been shown to significantly reduce the occurrence and severity of supragingival calculus formation.

Oral water irrigating devices

Several different types of water irrigation devices are on the market. They all use the principle of water under pressure to irrigate between and around the teeth to flush out debris. Some clinicians recommend the use of antimicrobial agents such as chlorhexidine rather than water. These devices are effective adjuncts to brushing, but they do not replace the action of the brush, since they are not known to remove tenaciously attached bacterial plaque. Oral irrigation has been shown to effectively reduce the severity of gingivitis and to remove loose food debris and nonadherent bacteria. However, it has not been shown to be effective in removing appreciable amounts of tenaciously attached, stainable dental plaque. If used according to manufacturers' directions, these devices will not traumatize the oral tissues. Injury to the soft tissues can be caused by excessive water pressure and improper placement of the tip.

The patient must be carefully instructed to follow directions. These devices should generally not be used to routinely rinse deep periodontal pockets because of the danger of forcing the bacteria out into the surrounding tissues. However, new equipment has been developed, and there is currently considerable interest in subgingival irrigation by the patient. More research is needed to determine the long-term effectiveness of this practice. Water irrigation devices are particularly effective cleaning aids for patients with orthodontic appliances and fixed prostheses.

Frequency of plaque control

Studies indicate that meticulous plaque removal every 24 to 48 hours is compatible with periodontal health. However, other research has shown improvement of periodontal health with frequency of plaque removal increased up to twice per day. Patients' needs and habits vary, but cleaning the teeth at least twice per day is recommended, with one session being particularly thorough.

Summary

Following is a summary of oral hygiene aids:

A. Primarily cleaning aids
    1. Toothbrush
        a. Manual
        b. Power-driven
    2. Disclosing tablets and solutions
    3. Dentifrices
    4. Mouthwashes and rinses
    5. Dental floss and tape
        a. Waxed
        b. Unwaxed
        c. Tufted
    6. Oral water irrigating devices
    7. Interproximal brushes
    8. Balsa wood wedge toothpicks
    9. Special toothpick and holder (Perio-Aid)
    10. Gauze strips, pipe cleaners, yarn
B. Primarily stimulating aids
    1. Rubber tip stimulator
    2. Balsa wood wedge toothpick

PLAQUE CONTROL PROGRAM

Several publications that deal entirely with plaque control programs are available. Each has its own philosophy, techniques, applications, approaches, and procedures. We recommend reading these publications to get a composite of the views and ideas in the area of plaque control programs. The plaque control program employed should be workable for both the patient and the dental personnel.

A plaque control program is designed to do the following:

1. Present useful knowledge to the patients about their dental disease and the purpose of plaque control in their individual oral health. The patients need to learn what they have to do.
2. Assist patients in learning and practicing new manual skills designed to attain and maintain their oral health. The patients need to learn how to control plaque accumulation.
3. Provide a series of experiences that will allow the patients to motivate themselves to use their knowledge and skills pertaining to oral hygiene on both a short- and a long-term basis.
4. Provide time to evaluate, reinforce, and support patients' skills, efforts, and successes.

Plaque control is most effective, and therefore more successful, if done before any other treatment is initiated. With this approach patients can experience the results of their own efforts and see that their periodontal health is within their control.

At the initial appointment an oral examination is performed to evaluate each patient's oral health and needs. At this time a diagnosis and treatment plan are established and accepted. If part of the treatment plan is the plaque control program, the program is presented to the patient. Its objectives, procedures, and commitments are explained to the patient as they relate to personal dental health needs. Participation in the program should be voluntary, since

health care maintenance is ultimately the patient's own responsibility.

Learning plaque control techniques

In the past an emphasis has been placed on strict plaque control programs in which all patients were requested to go through the same educational process regardless of their current skills, level of periodontal health, or interests. This method was effective in establishing a short-term improvement in plaque control, but the lack of individualization and long-term follow-up reduced the effectiveness of these concentrated oral hygiene programs.

We recommend that the learning sessions include experiences that allow the patients to learn at their own pace why and how they need to control their dental plaque. The lessons should be short in duration, present a limited amount of information in each session, provide early feedback on progress, be frequent until perfection is achieved, and be continued as needed during maintenance treatment. Some appointments can be devoted entirely to plaque control instructions, but reinforcement sessions should be combined with visits that include other therapeutic procedures. It is extremely important that each patient's individual needs, wants, and abilities be considered when selecting a method of teaching plaque control and the level of perfection expected. A total dental team (office) commitment to providing appropriate learning experiences for the patient creates a good motivational environment.

Plaque control room

The area in which the program is conducted should be as nonthreatening as possible. The majority of patients do not find the operatory and especially the dental chair conducive to relaxing; these often are stimuli for feelings of anxiety and fear. A special room or section of a room can provide a unique opportunity for learning in a relaxed, comfortable atmosphere. This room should contain all the motivational and educational tools necessary to facilitate the learning of new skills and information. It should also be equipped with sinks and proper lighting. A one-way mirror is an excellent learning device for students in educational settings. By using the mirror a student can observe a patient education session being conducted. Audiovisual equipment is also used for student feedback. The student can record the session and a critique can be conducted later.

Patient education

Before discussing the details of the plaque control program, certain guidelines for adult learning, motivation, and instructional methods need to be considered. These guidelines facilitate the learning transaction and increase the likelihood of changes in patient behavior.

The adult learner

Since the majority of plaque control program patients are adults, it is imperative that the nature of the adult learner be examined to facilitate teaching. Dental health educators need to understand the concepts of both teaching and learning. As adults, we require certain teaching techniques unique to adult learners.

In his book *The Adult Learner: A Neglected Species*, Malcolm Knowles describes four basic characteristics of the adult learner.

1. *Adults are self-directed.* This fact has certain implications for the dental health educator.
   a. The dental health educator cannot come across as dominant, judgmental, or superior.
   b. An environment of mutual inquiry and respect for the patient needs to be created.
   c. Adult patients need to be involved responsibly in setting their own objectives and outcomes. The decisions they make for themselves, whether approved by the dental health educator or not, need to be respected.
2. *Adults bring relevant experiences and*

knowledge into the learning situation. Ideal adult learning is not teacher-dominated and is not approached with the philosophy that the instructor has all the right answers for everyone.
   a. The knowledge and experiences of the patient need to be recognized because to ignore or invalidate an adult's knowledge is to ignore that patient as a person.
   b. Always solicit the patients' level of knowledge and skills before telling them something. The adult ego is easily wounded; adults react negatively to being told something they already know. By asking for information, the educator is both enhancing the patient's self-image and getting the benefit of what they know. Patients should be encouraged to contribute readily and to generate an exchange of ideas and attitudes.
   c. For learning to take place it is imperative that the educator create a climate that is supportive and encouraging. Adaptation, not learning, takes place in an environment that is noncaring, sarcastic, threatening, or indifferent.
3. *The adult learner is "now-oriented" and pragmatic.* Adult patients usually enter the plaque control program with the attitude, "If what I am learning does not have immediate application and usefulness, then I am not interested in taking the time or energy to learn it."
   a. Demonstrate to the patient how the information and skills to be learned are immediately applicable. How it works, how you can use it, and how you benefit, are the kinds of specific issues that need to be addressed.
4. *Adult learners are problem-solving-oriented.* Adults learn best if they perceive a need to learn or a need to solve a problem. This is also the essence of moti-

vational theory, which is addressed in the next section.

It is the responsibility of the educator to ensure that the patient is actively involved in the learning process. Allow and encourage the patient to demonstrate the skills and techniques being taught, as opposed to sitting passively observing the procedures.

Adults learn in a variety of ways. In designing the instructional situation, select materials that can be used individually or in small groups. Some patients like to study the material independently and ask questions as needed. Others want to socialize as they learn in an informal manner. Be flexible in the manner of presentation. Some people retain information better when it is presented orally, others when it can be read.

Patient motivation

Motivation is defined as factors within a person that stimulate, maintain, and channel behavior toward a goal. Dental health educators need to understand motivation so that they can be effective in eliciting productive action. It is important to understand that dental health educators cannot create motivation in others; they can only influence, stimulate, or help maintain it. When motivation is already high, the educator needs to provide direction and support to help patients reach their goals. When motivation is low, the educator's task is to clarify goals and stimulate a desire for change.

In attempting to motivate others, people often commit the following errors:

1. Trying to make people more motivated—remember, we cannot change others.
2. Assuming that one's own motivators also apply to others—patients may not value dental health at the same level as dental health professionals.
3. Failing to understand that people have numerous goals—dental health is only one of many patient goals, and it may have a low priority.
4. Disregarding others' needs to be involved in choosing and reaching their own goals—it is up to the patients to choose health, and their personal decisions need to be respected. It is the educator's responsibility to present the necessary information in a motivational context. It is the patient's responsibility to take that information and process and use it in a personal context. Individuals choose their own goals, so all motivation is self-motivation.

Motivation is the desire to satisfy needs and wants. A satisfied need or want is no longer a motivator. The key to motivation is for individuals to have goals or needs that are beyond their current positions (e.g., a healthy, stable periodontium). Creating a desire for change is the only reliable way to increase motivation. What is commonly known as motivation is really the process of illuminating needs and wants the person already has or stimulating new goals or wants by encouraging dissatisfaction with the present position. Dissatisfaction with the present situation leads to motivation.

Knowing what motivates others—which need is most motivating for a particular person in a particular situation—makes the dental health professional more successful in assisting patients. Although instruction is given only for a physical activity, actual long-term changes in behavior will depend on concurrent changes in thinking and feeling. For example, a patient with low self-esteem may not think it is important to worry about personal appearance. Understanding how to carry out a physical process that is recommended and the reasons for better dental hygiene does not mean that the process will become part of a daily routine. Until self-esteem improves, the patient will not make long-term behavioral change because it would serve no purpose.

Learning is also affected by changes in the individual over time. An instructional program should adapt to the patient's changing needs. As a person ages, physical coordination, dexterity, and speed decrease, but cognitive abilities do not. When new information is integrated into currently established cognitive structures, people of any age can learn.

In addition to physical changes, the adult is also undergoing role and status changes. The adult has many roles to play in life and each of these roles requires different responsibilities. The young adult's personal appearance and social life are usually great concerns; how will dental habits affect these factors? The parent of young children is usually more concerned about how dental habits will influence the family. The older adult may see dental hygiene as having impact on community and career status. For instance, you would approach a 40-year-old mother of seven differently than a 30-year-old ambitious male executive. The different stages of adult life bring with them different perspectives and, consequently, different needs.

It is important to recognize that adults are unique individuals with a rich history of personal experience. These experiences have created their identity and in doing so established their independence. Therefore when working with adults, it is important to keep the following ideas in mind:

1. Respect the values and experiences the patients bring to the learning situation.
2. Use those experiences in relating the new information to their current situation.
3. Incorporate active patient participation in all phases of the instructional process.

Implementing change

A change in behavior requires a change in attitude. The patient needs to be led through a series of attitude changes. First, the patient must become aware of the need for change. It is the responsibility of the educator to present information so that the patient can develop an understanding of the problem. With understanding, the patient will either dismiss the subject as unimportant or want more information. Ideally, the educator creates a sense of concern to which the patient responds by saying, "This is a problem that I need to solve. It is my responsibility, and making a change will benefit me."

Otherwise there will be no attitudinal change and therefore no behavioral change.

The following is a step-by-step summary for guiding patients toward change. It applies to any situation in which one person wants another to take action.

1. Awareness: Identify a need or problem (problem is periodontal disease)
2. Understanding: Explain the nature and extent of the problem (etiology of periodontal disease)
3. Concern: Show the consequences of the problem, and show that the client is responsible for making a change (consequences—advanced periodontal disease; prognosis—loss of tooth structure)
4. Dissatisfaction: Contrast the benefits of the program versus the cost of maintaining the present situation.
5. Action: Demonstrate and discuss how the program could be implemented to solve the problem.

To understand and influence patient's actions, first their attitudes must be understood—what motivates them as individuals. It is helpful to know patients well enough to reasonably predict how they will react to ideas.

Many of a patient's actions and attitudes are based on habit. Habits are ways people act without conscious thought or deliberate planning. These habits are initially shaped by experiences, beliefs, and conditioning, and they become routine and difficult to change. For patients to change habits, they must perceive a need.

Change needs to be implemented carefully. A gradual approach consists of a series of incremental steps, with short-term goals leading to a final goal. There are limits to the amount of change people can and will tolerate. When these limits are exceeded, people react strongly, and their productivity can drop. People accept change more readily if they perceive it as a small part of the total situation, and changes within tolerance limits can even stimulate people. For example, Measuring progress toward goals in the short term allows for maximum reinforcement and helps the patient view the change as manageable, heightening enthusiasm and confidence. Change should be carefully monitored and its effectiveness evaluated at each step.

Resistance to change

Resistance to change is not universal: people resist some changes, and people resist being changed. It is important to determine how much resistance exists and what the specific objectives are for each patient. Encourage and reinforce support for the change by emphasizing its benefits. The way a change is introduced may determine whether it is resisted. Be aware that initial enthusiasm may be temporary; therefore, reinforcement is essential.

Sometimes patients appear uncooperative, unproductive, and uncommitted. The educator needs to listen and observe to determine why patients are resistant. Is it attitude, need, or behaviorally oriented? Focus on both the facts presented and on any underlying emotional concern. Then respond by engaging in problem solving with the patient. The reaction to the patient's resistance is critical.

It is impossible to provide fixed rules on how to handle patient resistance. Much will be determined by the specific situation and the people involved.

Responding to the patients' concerns shows an interest in meeting their needs. This interest is the basis for service as health care professionals. If the resistance seems impossible to resolve, accept and respect the fact that it is the patient's right to choose a course of action.

The best way to reduce resistance is to create a desire for the change. Coercion, however, can lead to unpredictable reactions.

The designer of the instructional program must remember to adjust to the needs of each individual situation and keep the following ideas in mind:

1. Establish a nonthreatening learning atmosphere. This includes awareness of body language, tone of voice, and room arrangement. Many patients have had negative experiences in educational situations, and repeating such experiences may set almost insurmountable barriers to the learning process.

2. Be enthusiastic and convinced about the importance of plaque control. This will influence the patient.

3. Identify the patient's current skills. It is pointless to discuss flossing when the patient does not even brush.

4. Communicate with the patient as an equal. Never speak "down" to a patient. Patients come to the learning experience with a variety of skills and abilities and the instructor must be flexible enough to adjust the program accordingly. Do not use medical terms without explaining their meaning clearly and simply. Some patients are not comfortable asking for explanation.

5. Present an overview of the learning experience to the patient before beginning.

6. Orient the patient to the task at hand to give a clear understanding of what is involved. At the same time, limit the discussion of theory to what is needed to actually accomplish the task.

7. Present the material in small segments. Too much information at one time leads to confusion. It is more appropriate to give too little information than too much.

8. Speed of learning must be set by the patient. A patient should feel confident and be reasonably proficient at one skill before going on to another. This requires a great amount of patience. Do not expect a person to understand in one afternoon what professionals have studied for years.

9. The procedures should be performed on the patient's mouth. Instruction is most effective when the learner is actively involved.

10. Give the patient immediate feedback on each activity in a positive and reassuring manner.

11. Identify ways of measuring the successful attainment of the goals that are visible to both the instructor and the patient.

12. Evaluate on a continual basis. Evaluation should include not only the patient's progress but also the instructional process.

Remember that a person's ability to learn may be as much a consequence of social role and lifestyle as it is a consequence of intelligence. For actual changes in behavior to take place, instruction must be integrated with the patient's personal experiences and closely related to the patient's personal goals. Finally, all instructional activity must be flexible enough to adapt to the individual patient in each particular situation.

Scheduling appointments

Many diverse opinions exist on the correct timing for plaque control appointments. The number of appointments and time required may vary depending on the following:

1. Patient's level of motivation
2. Patient's physical dexterity, abilities, and competence
3. Patient's tissue state and oral hygiene conditions
4. Patient's attention span
5. Patient's dental IQ and background

More than one visit is needed for the patient to successfully learn essential information about plaque control. Usually several appointments are necessary to complete the instruction properly. The more visits for the purpose of training, the more likely it is that the patient will have a sustained result. The time lapse between sessions also varies. Four or five closely spaced visits, either daily or every other day if possible, are usually recommended. Close spacing of appointments allows for immediate feedback, checking on progress, and correction

of problems. Control or follow-up checks are an important aspect of the program. The first reevaluation should be scheduled 1 or 2 weeks after the initial instruction has been completed. Subsequent reevaluation and reinforcement should be continued during the active and recall phases of treatment if long-term results are to be achieved. The number of control checks depends on the needs of the individual patient. The primary purpose of the follow-up checks is to sustain motivation and to correct any techniques before causing damage to the tissues. The emphasis is on success through long-term motivation. Once the patient has completed the control checks a recall program is initiated.

Procedures in plaque control
First visit

1. Before any new skills are learned, the patient should understand and be given information about the following topics so the "why" of the skills to be learned is understood.
   a. What is dental plaque?
   b. How does dental plaque injure tissues?
   c. What does plaque look like in the mouth?
   d. How can plaque be removed?
   e. Depending on the patient's individual clinical situation, more extensive information may be exchanged, such as: What is a pocket? What is meant by bone loss?

   These questions are answered both verbally and nonverbally by demonstrating intraorally and/or by the use of audiovisual equipment. People learn more effectively by the stimulation of many senses—hearing, seeing, and doing.

2. The patient uses disclosing solution to visualize the plaque. If the liquid form is used, the patient is asked to swish the liquid vigorously in the mouth for approximately 30 seconds and then expectorate. To remove the excess stain, the

patient should rinse the mouth gently with water. If the tablet form is used, the patient should chew the tablet and swish the saliva vigorously in the mouth for about 1 minute. It is important to check that the solution has reached all parts of the mouth. If an area is missed, the patient must swish more vigorously. If the patient objects to the use of disclosing solutions, the colorless fluorescein solution and the Plaque-Lite can be used. With a good light and hand mirror the patient should observe the results. Show the patient the stained plaque.

3. If an oral hygiene index (OHI) (plaque index) is to be incorporated in the program, it should be taken immediately after the plaque has been disclosed. The OHI can have a twofold effect if used properly. First, it can serve as an excellent motivational device because the patient can see the results of plaque removal efforts. It also gives the patient a goal. Second, it serves as a record of the improvement or lack of improvement in the removal of plaque by the patient. The OHI records the number of teeth with plaque, and every surface with plaque (stained) is counted as "1." The oral hygiene index score is computed in percentage as follows:

$$\text{Oral hygiene index score (percent)} = \frac{\text{Number of teeth having plaque}}{\text{Total number of teeth present}} \times 100$$

The higher the score, the poorer the plaque removal. A score of zero indicates complete and total plaque removal. The OHI may be used at each visit or just at the first and last.

4. The phase microscope can be a valuable aid in patient motivation and education. By using the phase microscope, the patient can better understand the role of bacteria as etiological factors in gingival and periodontal disease. With the phase microscope the patient can actually see the living motile bacteria that have been removed from the dental plaque.

5. After the patient understands what plaque is and its role in periodontal disease, toothbrushing information can be given.
   a. Have the patient brush the teeth normally to remove the stained plaque.
   b. The teeth are restained and the effectiveness of the brushing is then evaluated by both the patient and the instructor. By observing areas not cleaned or insufficiently cleaned, the patient will recognize the inadequacy of the technique. At this point, care should be taken not to threaten or belittle the patient.
   c. Based on the patient's needs, a brushing technique and brush are selected. The toothbrushing technique should first be demonstrated on a dentiform model or study cast model and then in the mouth as the patient observes with a mirror. The patient then uses the brush as shown while the instructor guides, corrects, and offers suggestions. After the patient has completed brushing, the teeth should be restained so that the patient can see the more effective cleaning.

6. At the termination of the session the patient is given a toothbrush, disclosing tablets, appropriate literature, and a future appointment.

Second visit

1. After the first visit each session begins by checking on the progress and performance since the last visit. The patient discloses and demonstrates brushing ability. Corrections in technique are made at this time.
2. After the patient demonstrates a reasonable effectiveness in the use of the tooth-

brush, the dental flossing techniques are introduced. After brushing and disclosing the patient should view the plaque that usually remains on the interproximal surfaces. At this time the purpose of dental flossing is introduced. The patient is shown how to clean the proximal surfaces of the teeth. This can be done on a model first and then in the patient's mouth. The patient then uses the floss as the instructor guides, corrects, and offers suggestions. The teeth should be restained so that the patient can observe the effects of interproximal cleaning.

Subsequent appointments

Other special aids such as Stim-U-Dents and rubber tip stimulators should not be introduced until the patient has become reasonably proficient with both the toothbrush and dental floss. Supplemental aids should be kept as simple as possible. (Refer to the section on adjuncts to toothbrushing for details on their usage.)

Plaque control in the long-term maintenance of periodontal health

Repetition and reinforcement of plaque control techniques have been shown to be of significant value in improving oral hygiene performance over extended periods of time. In addition, regularly repeated professional tooth cleaning combined with toothbrushing instructions and fluoride applications have been shown to result in almost complete prevention of caries and periodontal disease. This study included professional appointments every 2 weeks for 2 years and every 4 to 8 weeks for 1 year. Using similar techniques, excellent results following periodontal surgery were also obtained.

The recommended time interval for performing professional scaling, root planing, prophylaxis, and plaque control reinforcement is quite variable depending on the effectiveness of the patient's oral hygiene, tendency to form calculus, and severity of the periodontal disease. Following active periodontal treatment it is recommended that the length of time between maintenance appointments be gradually increased until an interval is established that provides intervention before any periodontal health deterioration. The interval may vary from 1 month to 1 year.

Patient records

Records for each plaque control patient should be kept. These records are necessary for a personalized, organized, and effective program. These records tabulate each patient's progress and should be completed after each plaque control session. They should list areas of accomplishment, areas needing improvement, procedures started and completed, test results, and index scores. Any information that will help with patient care and instruction should also be included.

DIETARY COUNSELING IN PLAQUE CONTROL

Although local factors, especially dental plaque, have been isolated as the principal etiological factors of inflammatory periodontal disease, systemic factors may play a secondary or modifying role. One such systemic factor is nutritional deficiency. Although to date no evidence has shown that nutritional imbalances or deficiencies will alone cause periodontal pocket formation or periodontal disease, certain nutritional factors will influence the response of periodontal tissues to insults in the oral environment. Also, the physical character of the diet and the frequency and form of sugar exposures will influence bacterial growth and plaque formation.

Based on this evidence, it is important to consider the patient's dietary factors as a part of total patient care. In periodontal therapy dietary counseling has the following three basic objectives:

1. Reducing or eliminating the intake of refined sugars, especially sucrose

2. Maintaining a diet adequate in the essential nutrients
3. Ensuring a diet with sufficient intakes of foods of firm, fibrous texture

Two ways exist for the patient to reduce plaque formation. One method is to remove the plaque after it has formed by using the toothbrush and floss. The second method is to reduce the rate of its formation by lowering the intake of sweet (sucrose) foods and soft sticky foods.

Sugar intake

Oral bacteria use dietary sugars, in particular sucrose, for energy and synthesis of complex polysaccharides (glucans, levans, glycogen). When oral hygiene is poor, the consequence of dietary sugars is increased bacterial growth with the subsequent increased formation of local irritants and increased plaque formation. Current research indicates that frequent exposures to retentive sugars are most harmful, especially when they occur between meals. Therefore it is helpful to reduce exposures of retentive sugars and to eat them during meals if they are to be part of the patient's diet. The most common refined sugars include table sugar, molasses, honey, corn syrups, and corn sweeteners. Saccharin, aspartame (which contains aspartic acid, an amino acid), and sugar alcohols (mannitol and sorbitol) are acceptable substitutes for refined sugars.

Nutritionally adequate diet

Nutrients are the chemical substances in food that are needed by the body. A balanced diet is necessary for all the tissues of the body, including the periodontal tissues, to be properly nourished and to maintain optimal health. To obtain some information on the patient's dietary habits, a nutritional screening questionnaire (Fig. 12-17), a 24-hour recall (Fig. 12-18), or a 3- to 5-day diary or food record is helpful. Once this information is obtained, the patient's dietary intake can be analyzed and evaluated by using a simple and accurate guide, the basic

four food group plan (Fig. 12-19), or by a more specific method, computer nutrient analysis (Fig. 12-20). Computer diet analysis requires a nutrient data base that can be used on microcomputers or larger computer systems. The patient's diet record can also be sent to private or nonprofit organizations for complete computer analysis for a nominal fee.

Food texture and consistency

A diet composed of soft or sticky foods produces more plaque than a diet composed of firm, fibrous foods because soft sticky foods cling to the teeth and lead to the accumulation of debris. Firm, fibrous foods such as raw fruits and vegetables help clean away loose debris and provide stimulation to the tissues by means of the chewing process.

Dietary counseling procedures

Dietary counseling should be incorporated into the plaque control program when indicated. It is particularly necessary in patients with acute necrotizing ulcerative gingivitis. It is recommended that it be scheduled together with the plaque control sessions for optimal results in the control of plaque. The following components should be part of any diet counseling session:

1. Patient education. The patient needs to understand the role of nutrients in keeping a healthy periodontium and the role of sugars and soft, sticky foods in promoting bacterial growth and plaque formation. The diet counselor should develop an educational component tailored to the patient's level of interest, motivation, and understanding.
2. Dietary evaluation. Information on the patient's dietary intake must be analyzed and compared to a dietary standard or recommendation. After analysis and evaluation dietary modifications can be developed. It is important to use behavior modification counseling techniques that include patient involvement during the

Text continued on p. 179.

```
                        NUTRITIONAL SCREENING QUESTIONNAIRE*

Name _____ Date _____

Chart no. _____

1.  How many meals do you have a day? _____
    About what times are these eaten? _____

2.  Would you consider your appetite to be:
    _____ Good
    _____ Fair
    _____ Poor

3.  How often do you eat between meals?
    _____ Never
    _____ Occasionally
    _____ Often
    What foods do you usually eat between meals? _____
    _____

4.  How often do you drink soft drinks, fruit drinks ("Hi-C" or "Koolaid"), or
    any other sweetened beverages?
    _____ Never
    _____ Occasionally
    _____ Often _____(times/day)
    When do you drink these beverages?
    _____ With meals
    _____ Between meals
    _____ At both/either times

5.  How often do you drink coffee and/or tea?
    _____ Never
    _____ Occasionally
    _____ Often _____(cups/day)
    How do you drink your coffee/tea?  With:
    _____ Milk/Cream
    _____ Nondairy creamer
    _____ Sweetener _____
                    (Specify the kind.)

6.  How often do you use gum and/or mints?
    _____ Never
    _____ Occasionally
    _____ Often
    What brand do you use? _____

7.  How often do you use cough drops, throat lozenges, and/or antacid tablets?
    (Please circle which ones.)
    _____ Never
    _____ Occasionally
    _____ Often




*Adapted from DePaola, D., and Cheney, S.G.:  Preventive dentistry, Littleton,
Mass., PSG Publishing Co., 1979, p. 113.
```

FIGURE 12-17. Nutritional screening questionnaire. (Courtesy University of North Carolina, School of Dentistry.)   *Continued.*

NUTRITIONAL SCREENING QUESTIONNAIRE—continued

8. How often do you take vitamin or mineral supplements?
   ____ Never
   ____ Occasionally
   ____ Daily
   What is in your supplement? _____
   (Specify the type of vitamins or minerals.)

9. Are you presently on any special or restricted diet? Yes ___ No ___
   If so, what kind? _____

		Never	*Times/Day*	*Times/Week*
10.	a. How often do you eat/drink milk, cheese, yogurt, or other dairy foods?	____	____	____
	b. How often do you eat whole grain or enriched breads, cereals, or pasta?	____	____	____
	c. How often do you eat cooked or raw vegetables?	____	____	____
	d. How often do you eat/drink citrus fruit or juice (orange, grapefruit, tomato)?	____	____	____
	e. How often do you eat the following: carrots, pumpkin, sweet potatoes, greens, broccoli, spinach (or other dark yellow or green vegetable or fruit)?	____	____	____
	f. How often do you eat meat, fish, poultry, and eggs?	____	____	____
	g. How often do you eat peanut butter, nuts, dried peas or beans, or soybean products?	____	____	____
	h. How often do you eat your meals in restaurants or fast food places?	____	____	____

FIGURE 12-17, cont'd. Nutritional screening questionnaire. (Courtesy University of North Carolina, School of Dentistry.)

24-HOUR DIET EVALUATION

(Time)   FOOD INTAKE AND AMOUNT

_____   Breakfast

_____   Between meals

_____   Lunch

_____   Between meals

_____   Dinner

_____   Between meals

FOOD GROUPS

	Milk	Meat	Vegetable-fruit	Bread-cereal
Totals:				
Recommended				
Difference				

	Vitamin A intake	Vitamin C intake
Totals:		
RDA		
Difference		

SUGAR EXPOSURES

Form	During meal	Between meals	Totals
Sugar in solution (20 minutes/exposure)			
Solid and retentive sweets (40 minutes/exposure)			

Grand total   _____

Estimated time of acid exposure   _____

FIGURE 12-18. Twenty-four hour diet evaluation. (Courtesy University of North Carolina, School of Dentistry.)

DIET EVALUATION SUMMARY

(Patient) _____ (Date) _____

Food groups	Intake						Standard			Difference
	Day 1	Day 2	Day 3	Day 4	Day 5	Average per day	Child	Adolescent	Adult	
Milk group (milk, cheese)							3 to 4 servings	4 or more servings	2 servings	
Meat group (meat, fish, chicken, egg, dried peas, or beans)							2 or more servings			
Vegetable-fruit group							4 or more servings			
Vitamin C (mg)							45	50	60	
Vitamin A (RE)							400 to 700	800 to 1000	800 to 1000	
Bread-cereal group (enriched or whole grain)							4 or more servings			

Form	When eaten	Sweets intake					Total number of exposures	Total minutes of exposure
		Day 1	Day 2	Day 3	Day 4	Day 5		
Sugar in solution	During meal							
	End of meal							
	Between meals							
Solid and retentive sweets	During meal							
	End of meal							
	Between meals							

Total daily exposure: _____

Dr. _____

FIGURE 12-19. Diet evaluation summary. (Courtesy University of North Carolina, School of Dentistry.)

Nutrients	Your diet contains	Your diet should contain
Nutrients important for *tissue repair and healing*		
Zinc	14 mg	15 mg
Magnesium	514 mg	350 mg
Folic acid	314 μg	400 μg
Vitamin C	196 mg	60 mg
Protein	101 g	56 g
Nutrients important for *muscle development and function*		
Calcium	1499 mg	800 mg
Magnesium	514 mg	350 mg
Folic acid	314 μg	400 μg
Vitamin E	25 IU	10 IU
Protein	101 g	56 g
Nutrients for *bones and teeth*		
Calcium	1499 mg	800 mg
Phosphorus	2238 mg	800 mg
Magnesium	514 mg	350 mg
Fluoride	700 μg	1000 μg
Vitamin A	11298 IU	5000 IU
Vitamin C	196 mg	60 mg
Nutrients that can *increase resistance to infection*		
Vitamin A	11298 IU	5000 IU
Vitamin C	196 mg	60 mg
Protein	101 g	56 g

FIGURE 12-20. Diet analysis system. (From NUTRAN, Atlanta, Ga.)

analysis and evaluation processes. The patient should also participate in developing diet modifications. The diet modifications must be practical and realistic for the patient's lifestyle.

The Snyder test, an effective tool for patient motivation and education, can be incorporated into the dietary counseling sessions. The Snyder test is a colorimetric test that determines the acid products in metabolic activity by oral microorganisms (acidogenic bacteria) in a carbohydrate medium. This test evaluates the consumption of fermentable carbohydrates in the patient's diet. The acid production is evidenced by a change in color of the medium. The reading of the test should be done each day and the results recorded on the patient's record sheet. At least two tests should be performed on each patient, one at the beginning and one at the end of the program. A comparison of the two measures the improvement or lack of improvement in the patient's food and oral hygiene habits.

EQUIPMENT FOR PLAQUE CONTROL PROGRAM

1. Audiovisual and visual aids. These aids should be used selectively to introduce, demonstrate, and reinforce information and skills, but it is not advisable to substitute them for personal presentation and teaching.
   a. Projector and films
   b. Pamphlets and other reading material
   c. Flip charts and posters
   d. Models and study casts
   e. Slides
   f. Teaching machines
2. Mirrors
   a. Mouth
   b. Hand
   c. Wall

d. Illuminated magnifying
3. Light source (intraoral)
4. Sink and running water
5. Test materials and supplies
6. Phase microscope (not essential)
7. Dietary counseling materials (food diary); four food groups
8. Patient record sheet

PREVENTIVE PERIODONTICS

Plaque control is only one aspect of periodontal disease prevention. An effective recall system is an essential factor in preventive periodontics. The patient should be aware of the importance of regular dental visits as a preventive measure. The following procedures should be done at each recall visit, depending on the needs of the individual:

1. Regular and complete professional removal of hard and soft deposits on the teeth
2. Treatment of carious lesions with well-contoured restorations that facilitate rather than hinder plaque control
3. Correction of interproximal food impaction
4. Assessment of the need for orthodontic therapy to eliminate tooth crowding, improve axial loading of teeth, and provide a periodontal environment that is more resistant to inflammatory and traumatic destruction
5. Early replacement of missing teeth to prevent drifting and extrusion of teeth, which may predispose to plaque accumulation and occlusal trauma

SUGGESTED READINGS

Cross KP: Adults as learners, San Francisco, 1981, Jossey-Bass, Inc, Publishers.

Darkenwald G, and Merriam S: Adult education foundations of practice, New York, 1982, Harper & Row, Publishers, Inc.

Dental plaque slide series with text, Medicom, Inc., 1633 Broadway, New York, NY 10019.

Developing a plaque control program. Produced by the Section on Instructional System Design, Division of Peri-

odontology, School of Dentistry, University of California, San Francisco, Berkeley, Calif, 1972, Praxis Publishing Co.

Emler BF, et al: The value of repetition and reinforcement in improving oral hygiene performance, J Periodontol 51:228, 1980.

Gould R: Transformations, New York, 1978, Simon & Schuster, Inc.

Grossman E, et al, Six-month study of the effects of a chlorhexidine mouthrinse on gingivitis in adults, J Periodont Res Suppl 33-43, 1986.

Kidd JR: How adults learn, 1973, New York, Associated Press.

Kornman DS: The Role of supragingival plaque in the prevention and treatment of periodontal diseases, J Periodont Res Suppl 5-22, 1986.

Loe J, and Schiott CR: The effect of mouth rinses and topical application of chlorhexidine in the development of gingivitis in man, J Periodont Res 5:79, 1970.

Loe H, Theilade E, and Jensen SB: Experimental gingivitis in man, J Periodontol 36:177, 1965.

Newburn E: Chemical and mechanical removal of plaque. In the compendium of continuing education in dentistry, Supplement No. 6, 1985.

Nizel A: Nutrition in preventive dentistry: science and practice, Philadelphia, 1972, WB Saunders Co, pp 303-491.

Nonsurgical antibacterial approaches to periodontal treatment, JADA 116:23-32, 1988.

Nyman S, Lindhe J, and Rosling B: Periodontal surgery in plaque infected mouths, J Clin Periodontol 4:240-249, 1977.

Perspectives on oral microbial therapeutics, Littleton, Mass, 1987, PSG Publishing Co, Inc.

Rees TD, Orth CF: Oral ulcerations with use of hydrogen peroxide, J Periodontol 57:689-692, 1986.

Rosling B, et al: The healing potential of the periodontal tissues following different techniques of periodontal surgery in plaque-free dentitions, J Clin Periodontol 3:233-250, 1976.

Sanz M, et al: A comparison of the effect of a 0.12% chlorhexidine gluconate mouthrinse and placebo on post periodontal surgical therapy, J Dent Res (abstract), March 1987.

Sheehy G: Passages New York, 1973, Elsevier-Dutton Publishing Co, Inc.

Smith R: Learning how to learn, Chicago, 1982, Cambridge Books.

Youngblood JJ, et al: Effectiveness of a new home plaque-removal instrument in removing subgingival and interproximal plaque: a preliminary in vivo report, The Compendium of Continuing Education in Dentistry, Suppl No. 6, 1985

Zacherl WA, et al: The effect of soluble pyrophosphates on dental calculus in Adults, JADA 110:737-738, 1985.

CHAPTER 13

Basic Instrumentation for Scaling and Root Planing

Scaling and root planing are the clinical procedures for removing all calculus and softened tooth structure to achieve a smooth, hard surface. *Scaling* is the process by which calculus is removed from the tooth surface. On enamel, scaling is usually adequate to completely remove the calculus deposit. This is because the attachment of the calculus to enamel is relatively superficial; the calculus is not deeply embedded into surface irregularities. *Root planing* consists of meticulously removing small deposits of calculus and softened cementum or dentin from the root surface to render it smooth and hard. This procedure is necessary to adequately remove calculus that is deeply enmeshed into the surface irregularities of cementum. Scaling alone is not usually sufficient to completely remove calculus deposits attached to the root surface. Root smoothness is advantageous because rough surfaces collect and retain plaque more readily. In addition, recent evidence indicates that cementum exposed to plaque, calculus, and a pocket environment becomes permeated with toxic substances such as endotoxins, which can be a source of irritation to the gingiva. Root planing has been shown to be effective in reducing these toxic products in the root. To ensure maximum removal of the irritants, a portion of the cementum is usually removed.

In summary, even though calculus is considered a secondary etiologic factor, its removal is important in the control of periodontal disease. This is because calculus holds the bacterial plaque in close contact with the gingival tissues. Recent studies indicate that the clinician's ability to completely remove calculus from root surfaces in deep pockets is limited with the nonsurgical approach. However, this should not discourage the operator from trying to achieve perfection in this procedure. Therapeutic studies have shown that scaling and root planing when combined with effective oral hygiene and regular periodontal maintenance therapy can be effective in the treatment of gingivitis and early to moderate periodontitis.

Instruments are designed for specific purposes in scaling and root planing. The instruments used for these procedures are classified into five basic categories according to their unique functions:

1. Sickle scalers
2. Hoes
3. Files
4. Chisels
5. Curets

Although dental explorers and periodontal probes are not designed for calculus removal or smoothing root surfaces, they both play an important role in the removal process and therefore deserve mention.

Explorers are delicate instruments designed and primarily used to detect caries and other tooth irregularities such as calculus deposits, root roughness, anatomical defects, and margins of restorations. Explorers come in a vari-

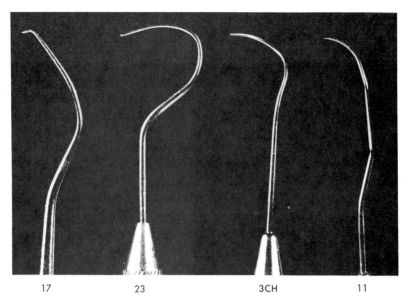

17   23   3CH   11

FIGURE 13-1. Typical explorer tips used to detect calculus and irregularities on tooth surfaces. From left to right, numbers 17, 23, 3 CH, and 11.

ety of shapes, sizes, and working ends. Some are best suited for caries detection and others for the detection of fine subgingival irregularities. Numbers 17, 23, 3CH, and 11-12 explorer tips are recommended for the detection of subgingival calculus (Fig. 13-1). The explorer should be used before scaling and root planing are performed to locate deposits and after these procedures are done to check for smoothness of the tooth surface and effectiveness of removal (Fig. 13-11, *A* and *D*).

Like the explorer the *periodontal probe* (Fig. 11-12) is also used for examining and evaluating the oral tissues. It is not used for caries detection, since it does not have a sharp point for retention in carious areas. Probes that are noted for their delicate design can be used for detection of root irregularities and hard deposits. The periodontal probe's primary function is to measure the depth of the gingival sulcus or periodontal pocket. The probe's unique feature is its millimeter calibrations for measurement.

PARTS OF THE INSTRUMENT

All hand instruments consist of three basic sections: the handle, the shank and the working end (Fig. 13-2). The *handle* is the part of the instrument grasped by the operator. Handles are available in a variety of sizes, shapes, and surface textures. The handle selected should be wide enough to provide for a comfortable grasp to prevent muscular fatigue. Ribbed or textured handles provide for easy gripping and less slippage. Hollow handles as opposed to solid handles allow for greater tactile perception and are lighter in weight.

The *shank* is that portion of the instrument that connects the working end with the handle. The shanks of instruments vary in both angle (straight or curved) and length. The particular angle and length are designed for access in particular areas and specific tooth surfaces according to the location, depth, and amount of calculus deposits. Shank shape, length, and strength selection are extremely important for effective

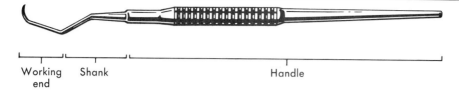

Working   Shank   Handle
end

FIGURE 13-2. Dental curette illustrating the basic parts of a hand instrument: working end, shank, handle.

and efficient removal of deposits from the teeth.

The *working end* is that part of the instrument that contacts the tooth and performs the actual work. Instruments are classified based on the unique design of the working end. Some types of instruments are manufactured with replaceable tips that screw into a separate handle (cone-socket tips).

Instruments can be purchased with one working end; these are referred to as single-ended instruments. Double-ended instruments have two working ends, which are located on each end of the handle. These two working ends are usually paired (mirror images of each other) or complementary.

INSTRUMENT GRASP

The way an instrument is held is important in terms of instrument stability, control, and effectiveness. Generally the following are the three basic ways to hold periodontal instruments:

1. Standard pen grasp (Fig. 13-3)
2. Modified pen grasp (Fig. 13-4)
3. Palm and thumb grasp (Fig. 13-5)

Standard pen grasp

With the standard pen grasp the instrument is held between the tips of the thumb and the index fingers on one area of the handle with the side of the middle finger closer to the shank of the instrument. This grasp does not provide maximum stability; the instrument tends to rotate between the grasping fingers when applying pressure to the blade.

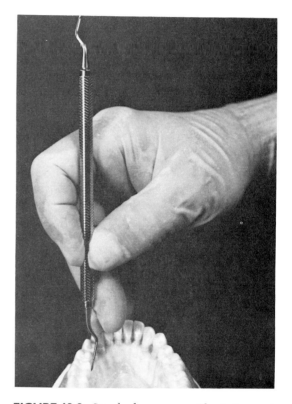

FIGURE 13-3. Standard pen grasp. The instrument is braced against the side of the middle finger.

Modified pen grasp

With the modified pen grasp the pad rather than the side of the middle finger is used. It is also suggested that placing the index finger slightly farther away from the shank than the thumb adds stability. This creates three points of contact rather than the two in the standard pen grasp. The modified pen grasp is consid-

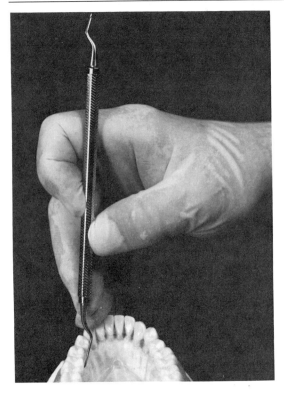

FIGURE 13-4. Modified pen grasp. The instrument is braced against the pad of the middle finger, which is also being used as the fulcrum or finger rest.

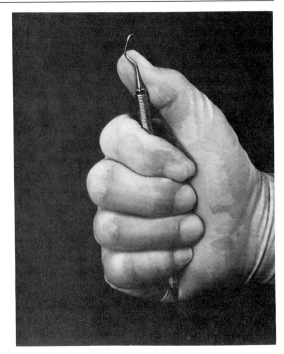

FIGURE 13-5. Palm grasp. The instrument is braced against the thumb.

ered the most desirable method of holding periodontal instruments.

Palm and thumb grasp

The palm and thumb grasp can be utilized to generate strong forces, but is considered the least desirable grasp because of decreased flexibility and tactile sensitivity. With this technique the handle of the instrument is held in the palm of the hand with the fingers grasping the handle. The thumb is then placed at the junction of the shank and handle for control. Because this is considered a power grasp, it can be useful in removing heavy, tenacious calculus. It is also useful when holding an instrument for sharpening in a handpiece.

FINGER REST (FULCRUM)

Regardless of the holding method selected, a finger rest should be used at all times when the instruments are being used. A finger rest is essential for instrument control and stability, and it facilitates proper movement of the instrument for efficient removal of deposits. Without control the instrument can slip, causing tissue laceration and injury to the patient (Fig. 13-4). An ideal finger rest provides a stable fulcrum point, allows proper blade angulation to the tooth, and facilitates the wrist-forearm motion to mobilize the instrument.

Principles of establishing a finger rest

1. Pad of the ring finger should be used for the finger rest.
2. Finger rest should be within the mouth on solid tooth surface or surfaces when-

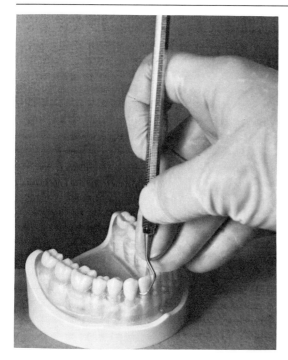

FIGURE 13-6. Ideal fulcrum with ring finger on central incisors adjacent to the lateral incisor being instrumented.

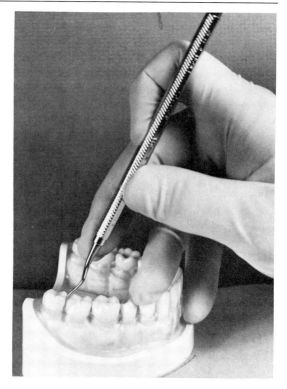

FIGURE 13-7. Fulcrum on the first premolar, which is distant from the second molar being instrumented.

ever possible. Finger rests outside the mouth (lips, chin, cheeks), while sometimes necessary, are inadvisable because these areas are mobile and slippage is possible. Also, the patient usually finds extraoral rests uncomfortable.

3. Tooth surface used for a rest should be kept as dry as possible to prevent slippage.

4. Finger rest should be on teeth as close as possible to the working area, preferably the adjacent teeth in the same arch (Fig. 13-6).

Variations in finger rests

In some areas of the mouth anatomical limitations prevent the establishment of an ideal fulcrum rest on an adjacent tooth. The following are examples of modified fulcrums that can be utilized in these situations:

1. Fulcrum on a tooth distant from the tooth being instrumented (Fig. 13-7).
2. Fulcrum in the opposite arch (Fig. 13-8).
3. Fulcrum on a finger of the opposite hand (Fig. 13-9).
4. Cross-arch fulcrum (Fig. 13-10).
5. Extraoral fulcrum on the chin. This is most commonly utilized when instrumenting the maxillary posterior teeth.
6. Stabilization of instrument with finger(s) from opposite hand when compromised fulcrums are utilized.

SUBGINGIVAL SCALING AND ROOT PLANING INSTRUMENTATION

Effective subgingival scaling and root planing are more difficult procedures to perform than

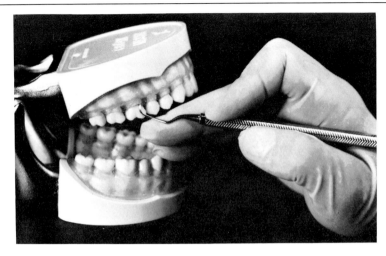

FIGURE 13-8. Fulcrum on the mandibular anterior teeth to instrument the maxillary first molar.

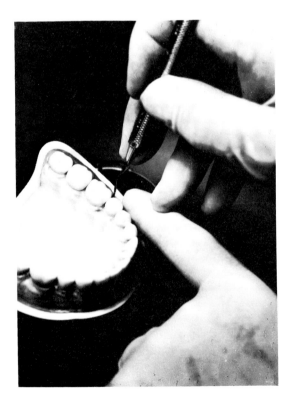

FIGURE 13-9. Fulcrum established on the index finger of the opposite hand.

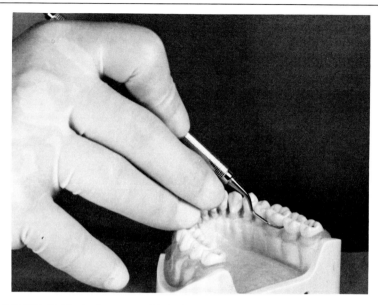

FIGURE 13-10. Fulcrum established on the opposite side of the same arch.

supragingival scaling. Factors that make them more challenging are harder, more tightly attached calculus; a soft-tissue covering that inhibits access, prevents visibility, and forces the operator to rely heavily on tactile sensitivity to detect calculus and root roughness; and more complex instruments designed to reach into deep pockets and adapt to specific root surfaces. The methods of using the different types of instruments are discussed in the next section of this chapter, but the following suggestions are applicable to root planing regardless of the instruments used:

1. Prior to instrumentation subgingival calculus or root irregularities should be located with a dental explorer used with a light, delicate stroke (Fig. 13-11, *A*).

2. Following the establishment of a stable finger rest, the periodontal instrument is carefully inserted to the base of the pocket. Light strokes will detect calculus deposits; when these are found, the instrument should be moved apically over the calculus until the most apical level of the calculus is noted. Usually a distance of 0.2 to 1 mm is found between the apical edge of the calculus and the bottom of the pocket (Figs. 13-11, *B*, and 13-12).

3. Pressure is then applied laterally against the tooth surface to ensure instrument control, tactile sensitivity, and minimal soft-tissue trauma. A series of controlled, short, overlapping strokes are used to remove the calculus. The initial strokes involve considerable pressure. However, as the calculus is crushed and removed, gradually lighter and more meticulous movements are employed. The operator may also choose to use a smaller, more delicately constructed instrument to facilitate tactile sensitivity for the final root planing procedures (Fig. 13-11, *C*).

4. Instrumentation should continue until the root surface is smooth and hard.

5. Entire root surface in the pocket should be planed, being sure to instrument all concavities and involved furcation areas.

6. Using a dental explorer with a delicate

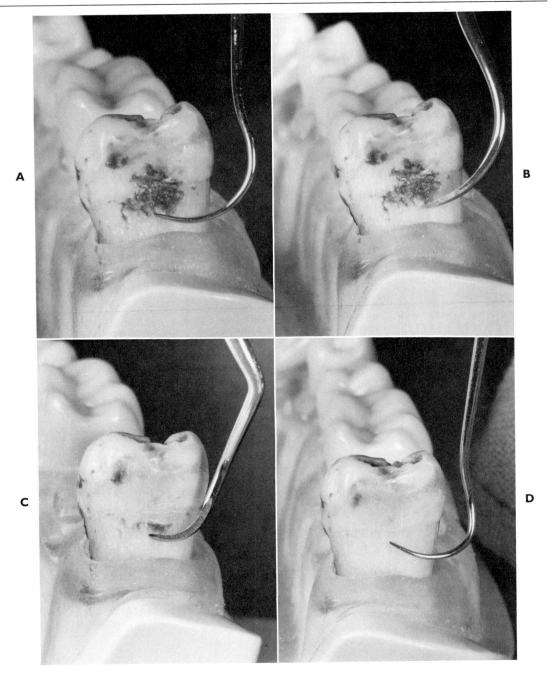

FIGURE 13-11. **A,** Detecting calculus with a 3CH explorer tip. **B,** Removal of heavy calculus with a McCall 17S universal curet. **C,** Removal of residual calculus and root planing with a Gracey curet. **D,** Checking the smoothness of the tooth surface following the scaling and root planing.

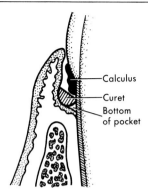

FIGURE 13-12. Curet positioned to remove subgingival calculus.

stroke, the entire root surface is examined for residual calculus, root roughness, and surface hardness (Fig. 13-11, *D*). A more detailed explanation of the instrumentation is found in the discussion of curets (pp. 191-197).

SICKLE SCALER
Characteristics

The sickle scaler is an instrument with two straight cutting edges. These cutting edges are formed by the convergence of the facial surface and the two lateral surfaces, which come together to form a sharp, pointed tip. The cross section of the blade is triangular in shape (Fig. 13-13). Some sickles are produced with backs that are flattened, thus eliminating the pointed tip. Two types of sickle scalers are available: straight sickle and curved or contra-angled sickle. These are identical in the working end, but the contra-angle has a curved shank so that it can be adapted to the posterior teeth, and the straight sickle has a straight shank for use on the anterior teeth or bicuspid area if proper angulation can be maintained.

Uses

1. To remove supragingival calculus, primarily.
2. To remove calculus just below or adjacent to the gingival margin only when

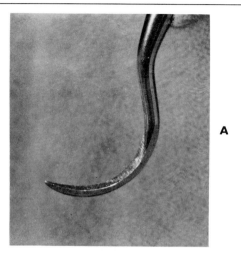

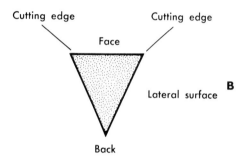

FIGURE 13-13. A, Typical sickle scaler. **B,** Cross section of the working end of a sickle scaler.

the tissue is flexible enough to insert the scaler without damaging the tissue. The sickle should not be inserted deeply into the sulcus or pocket because the sharp tip will lacerate the soft tissue and the straight cutting edges cannot be adapted to the curved contours of the tooth.

Utilization

1. Blade is placed on the tooth in such a way that the angle between the face of the instrument and the tooth surface is less than 90 degrees but not less than 45 degrees (Fig. 13-14).
2. Instrument is used with a pull stroke.

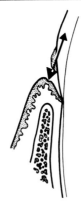

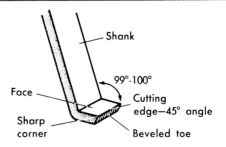

FIGURE 13-15. Hoe scaler.

FIGURE 13-14. Cross section illustrating a sickle scaler properly positioned to remove supragingival calculus.

HOE
Characteristics

The hoe is a scaler with one straight cutting edge that is formed by the union of the face of the instrument and the beveled toe of the blade. This union also forms two sharp corners on the sides of the cutting edge (Fig. 13-15). The shank of a hoe comes with various angulations to gain access to different areas of the mouth and tooth surfaces. Hoes may be purchased as single- or double-ended instruments.

Uses

1. To remove heavy, gross supragingival calculus.
2. To remove heavy, gross calculus slightly below or adjacent to the marginal gingiva only if the tissue is flexible enough to permit easy insertion. Care must be taken when inserting the hoe slightly below the gingival margin. One sharp corner can gouge the root surface, and the other can lacerate the sulcular epithelium. Rounding the corners of the cutting edge with a sharpening stone before use will prevent this trauma.
3. To remove calculus on buccal and lingual surfaces; also used on proximal surfaces adjacent to endentulous areas.

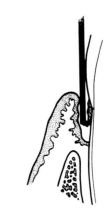

FIGURE 13-16. Cross section illustrating a hoe scaler properly positioned to remove subgingival calculus.

Utilization

1. Entire cutting edge is placed on the tooth surface. To ensure proper leverage, stability, and control, the shank should be positioned, if possible, so it contacts the tooth surface. Before activation the shank should be as parallel to the long axis of the tooth as possible (Fig. 13-16).
2. Hoe is used with a pull stroke in a vertical direction toward the occlusal or incisal surface.

CHISEL
Characteristics

The chisel is a scaler with one straight, flat, beveled cutting edge and a blade that is continuous with a slightly curved shank. As with the

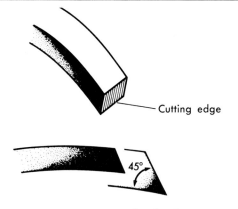

FIGURE 13-17. Chisel scaler.

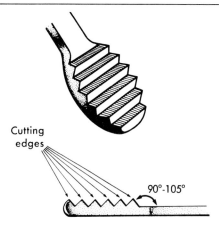

FIGURE 13-18. Periodontal file.

hoe, sharp corners are formed on both sides of the cutting edge (Fig. 13-17).

Uses

The chisel is used to remove heavy supragingival calculus from the proximal surfaces of anterior teeth when the embrasure spaces are open.

Utilization

1. Entire working end is placed on the tooth so that the sharp points do not nick or gouge the tooth surface.
2. Push with horizontal stroke in buccal to lingual direction to dislodge the calculus on the proximal surfaces.

FILE
Characteristics

The file has multiple cutting edges similar to those of a hoe. The base of the blades can be round, oval, or rectangular extensions of the base (Fig. 13-18). The shanks of files vary in angulation and length for proper adaptation to tooth surfaces.

Uses

1. To remove heavy, gross supragingival calculus.
2. To remove gross calculus slightly below or adjacent to the gingival margin only if

the tissues are flexible enough for easy insertion.
3. To remove calculus by fracturing, crushing, or fragmenting the deposits. This allows for easier removal with the curet.
4. To smooth the cementoenamel junction of the tooth surface.
5. To remove overhanging margins of dental restorations.

Utilization

1. The entire working surface should be placed flat against the tooth surface to avoid tissue trauma and gouging the root surface. Adaptation of the straight cutting edges to the curved surfaces is difficult.
2. For stability and control, the shank, if possible, should rest against the tooth surface (Fig. 13-19).
3. The file is activated with a pull stroke.

CURET
Characteristics

The curet is an instrument with one or two cutting edges on a spoon-shaped working end. The cutting edges are curved, and the back of the instrument is rounded (Fig. 13-20, *A* and *B*). The advantage of this design is that when the instrument is inserted beneath the gingival

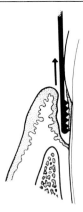

FIGURE 13-19. Cross section illustrating a periodontal file properly positioned to remove subgingival calculus.

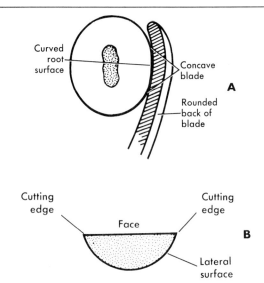

FIGURE 13-20. A, Curved surface of a curet positioned against the convex root surface. **B,** Cross section of the working end of a curet.

margin it will conform closely to the root contours and cause minimal laceration of the soft-tissue wall of the pocket (Fig. 13-20, A, and 13-12). The absence of sharp corners and pointed tips on the blades minimizes gouging of the root surfaces. These features along with the relatively small size and delicate tactile sensitivity make the instrument excellent for subgingival scaling and root planing.

There are two basic types of curets used for scaling and root planing. The universal curets have two cutting edges, and the face of the blade is usually perpendicular to the lower shank (Fig. 13-21). Various shank designs and the double cutting edges enable these curets to be used in different areas in the mouth. The area-specific curets, such as the Gracey curets, are designed to work on specific surfaces of certain teeth. They are provided in sets; right and left paired instruments are required to properly instrument an entire dentition (Fig. 13-22). These curets have only one cutting edge, and the face of the blade is positioned at a 70-degree angle rather than a 90-degree angle to the lower shank of the instrument (Fig. 13-23). The cutting edge is the one farthest from the instrument handle, or the lower edge of the blade. This feature enables the clinician

to achieve the proper angle of the blade to the tooth subgingivally by making the lower shank of the instrument parallel to the long axis of the tooth (Fig. 13-24, A and B). With the universal curet the shank must be tilted slightly toward the tooth surface being instrumented to achieve a less than 90° angle between the blade and the tooth (Fig. 13-25). This is considered optimal for effective scaling and root planing.

Curets also vary according to the size of the blade and the thickness of the shank. Larger curets are used to remove heavy subgingival deposits, and smaller curets are used for fine scaling and root planing (Fig. 13-11, B and C).

Utilization

The following is a series of steps to be taken when performing a subgingival scaling and root planing procedure with curets:

1. Sterilize the instruments needed for the entire procedure on a tray or separate container. Instruments should be placed on a sterile surface for use during the procedure. Techniques should be em-

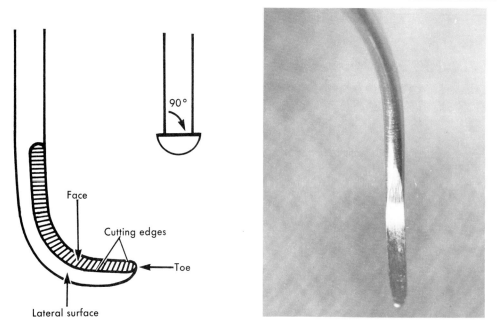

FIGURE 13-21. Typical universal curet with two cutting edges and a blade at a 90-degree angle to the lower shank.

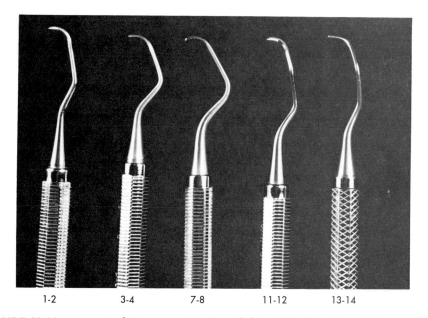

| 1-2 | 3-4 | 7-8 | 11-12 | 13-14 |

FIGURE 13-22. Five paired Gracey curets. From left to right: the 1-2 and 3-4 are used on anterior teeth, and the 7-8, 11-12, and 13-14 are used on posterior teeth.

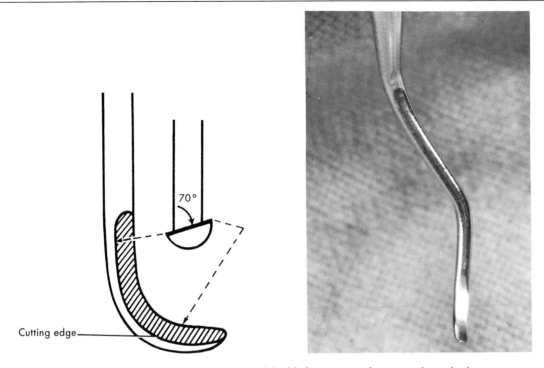

FIGURE 13-23. Area-specific curet. Face of the blade is at a 70-degree angle to the long axis of the shank. The cutting edge, which is curved, is the lowest edge of the blade.

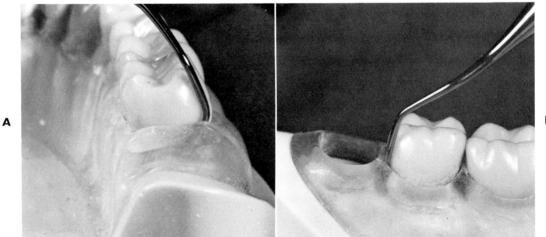

FIGURE 13-24. **A,** Lower shank of Gracey curet parallel with the long axis of the tooth from the buccolingual perspective. **B,** Lower shank of Gracey curet parallel with the long axis of the tooth from the mesiodistal perspective.

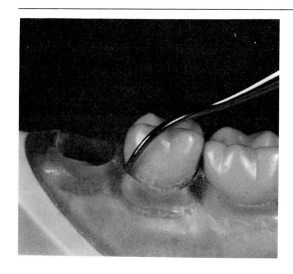

FIGURE 13-25. Mesial tilting of a universal curet to achieve the proper 70-degree angle of the blade to the tooth.

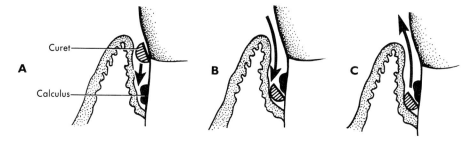

FIGURE 13-26. A, Insertion of curet with face of blade approximately parallel to the long axis of the tooth. **B,** Rotation of blade to be more than 45 degrees but less than 90 degrees to the root. **C,** Vertical movement of the curet to remove the calculus.

ployed to insure maximum protection from infectious diseases. The clinician and assistants should wear surgical gloves and protective eyewear and masks. The dental chair and unit should be disinfected and barrier materials placed where appropriate.

2. Obtain adequate local anesthesia with topical or injected anesthetics as required.

3. Using a light explorer and compressed air, determine the location of the subgingival calculus deposits (Fig. 13-11, *A*).

4. Grasp the curet with the modified pen grasp (Fig. 13-4).

5. Establish an appropriate fulcrum (Fig. 13-6).

6. With the face of the blade parallel to the long axis of the tooth, gently insert the instrument into the pocket until the cutting edge is apical to the calculus deposit (Fig. 13-26, *A*).

7. Change the angle of the blade to the tooth surface so that it is more than 45 degrees but less than 90 degrees (Fig. 13-26, *B*).

8. Exert firm lateral forces against the

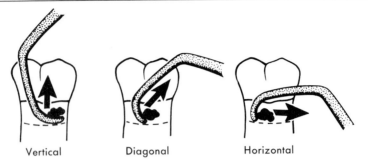

FIGURE 13-27. Different stroke directions to dislodge calculus.

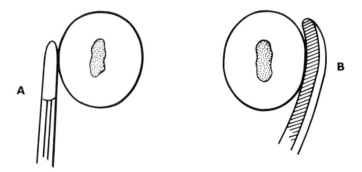

FIGURE 13-28. Adaptation of curet blade to tooth surface. **A,** Open angle with minimal contact between the tooth and the instrument. **B,** Closed angle, allowing closer adaptation of blade to the convex tooth surface.

tooth surface with a series of short, controlled, overlapping strokes. Vertical, diagonal, or horizontal strokes can be made by wrist-forearm rotation (Fig. 13-26, *C* and 13-27, *A* to *C*).

9. When the calculus is on the root surface, planing is usually required to completely remove it and achieve maximum smoothness. The root planing instrumentation is done with light but firm lateral pressure and a sequence of long, overlapping strokes until a smooth, hard surface is achieved. Maximum adaptation of the blade to the tooth surface should be maintained during the procedure (Fig. 13-28, *A* and *B*). This often requires rotation of the instrument to

accommodate the concavities, convexities, and line angles of root surfaces (Fig. 13-29, *A* to *C*).

10. Rinse and debride the instrumented areas.

11. Give appropriate posttreatment instructions to the patient.

a. The teeth and soft tissues may be painful following the procedure. Rinse with warm water, a commercially available or prescribed mouthwash, and take an analgesic as required. You should be able to resume use of a toothbrush and dental floss within 24 hours.

b. Minimal bleeding from the tissues is normal, but if it is excessive or persistent, telephone the office.

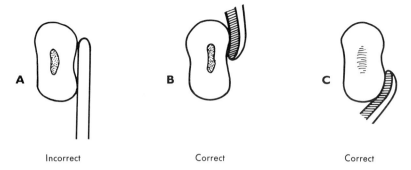

FIGURE 13-29. A, Incorrect adaptation of curet to concave root surface. **B,** Correct rotation of curet to allow rounded end to plane concavity. **C,** Placement of curet to adapt the blade to the convex surface of the line angle.

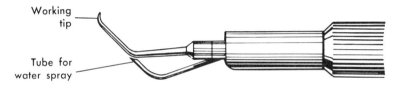

FIGURE 13-30. Typical ultrasonic scaling instrument.

c. The teeth may be sensitive to temperature changes following the procedure. This is usually temporary, resolving itself if the teeth are effectively brushed and cleaned.

d. Contact the dentist at the office or at home if any unusual difficulties arise following the treatment.

12. Reappoint the patient for treatment of another area of the mouth. When all areas of the mouth are completed, reappoint the patient for a periodontal reevaluation. This should be done no sooner than 2 weeks but preferably within about 2 months.

ULTRASONIC DEVICES
Characteristics

Ultrasonic devices work on the principle of high-frequency energy vibrations. These vibrations move the instrument tip in a back-and-forth motion at approximately 25,000 cycles per second with a length of approximately 0.001 inch. The energy vibrations remove the deposits by fracturing them.

Ultrasonic vibrations produce large amounts of heat, and this heat can cause damage to both the tooth and the tissues. A cooling system of water is incorporated into the unit to eliminate the effects of the heat. The water also can flush out the sulcus area. A saliva ejector or aspirator must be used to eliminate the water. A typical ultrasonic scaling instrument is shown in Fig. 13-30.

Uses

1. To remove calculus, stain, and debris; most effective with heavy, gross amounts of deposits and stain and usually require less effort and time than manual hand instrument removal.

2. To assist in soft tissue curettage and periodontal surgery.

3. To remove deposits when tissues are hy-

persensitive, as in acute gingival conditions such as necrotizing ulcerative gingivitis, because less tissue insult occurs.

4. To remove overhanging margins on amalgam restorations.
5. To remove excess cement in orthodontic procedures.

Controversy exists over the effectiveness of the ultrasonic instruments as compared with scalers and curets in removal of calculus, root planing, and resolution of periodontal disease. While recent studies show ultrasonic instrumentation to be effective in arresting progressive periodontitis, many clinicians still depend heavily on the curets to achieve maximum root preparation.

Utilization

1. Use short, rapid, vertical or oblique strokes.
2. Use light pressure with a featherlike touch.
3. Tip or lateral surface of the instrument must be in contact with the deposit for it to be dislodged.
4. Tip should be kept in constant motion and never remain stationary for too long.
5. Instrument tip should be blunt, not sharp and pointed, to avoid damaging the root surface.
6. Proper instrument tip should be used for maximal efficiency in removal of deposits. A variety of tips are available.

Care must be taken to use the device correctly because improper use may produce gouging, scratching, and roughening of the root surface.

CARE OF INSTRUMENTS

1. Using heavy rubber gloves, all instruments should be washed and scrubbed thoroughly to remove all blood and debris following their use.
2. All instruments should be sterilized and packaged to preserve sterility until used. During treatment the instruments should be kept on a previously sterilized surface when not in use.
3. Instruments should be sharpened at the first sign of dullness. Instruments need to be sharpened between each procedure as well as during the scaling and root planing. If a sharpening stone is sterilized with each instrument kit, the sharpening can be done without breaking the sterility chain.

INSTRUMENT SHARPENING

Instruments must be sharp for effective and efficient scaling and root planing. Dull instruments not only increase working time and physical effort but also can burnish the calculus rather than removing it and cause tissue trauma as well. Sharpening is the process of planing the surfaces of the instrument that form the cutting edge of the blade until a fine cutting edge is restored without losing the original angles and design of the instrument.

Sharpening stones

Instrument sharpening is done with stones. The stones used are composed of masses of minute abrasive crystal particles that grind the dull blade. Sharpening stones are available in various grits, designs, and textures.

Two general types of stones are available as follows:

1. Mounted stones. Cylindrical stones that come in a variety of sizes and are mounted for use in a slow-speed handpiece (Fig. 13-31, A).
2. Unmounted stones.
   a. Flat stones. Rectangular stones that are either flat or have a grooved surface for sharpening instruments with curved blades (Fig. 13-31, B).
   b. Rounded stones. Cylindrical or rectangular stones with rounded edges (Fig. 13-31, C).

The design of the sharpening stone selected will depend upon the shape of the instrument cutting edge as well as the surface of the blade

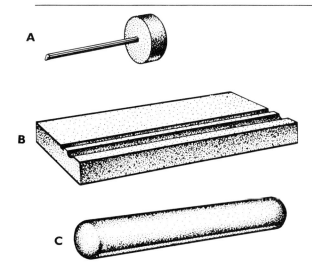

FIGURE 13-31. Sharpening stones. **A,** Mounted sharpening stone to be used in a slow-speed handpiece. **B,** Flat sharpening stone with grooves. **C,** Cylindrical sharpening stone.

to be planed. A flat stone is used to sharpen straight cutting edges such as those found on scalers, hoes, and chisels (Figs. 13-36, 13-37, 13-38). It is also used to sharpen a curet when the lateral surfaces of the blade are being planed (Fig. 13-40, *A* to *C*). Stones with rounded surfaces are most often used to plane the face of the curet blade (Fig. 13-32, *A* and *B*). The mounted stones can be used to sharpen the face or the lateral surfaces of scalers or curets (Fig. 13-33). Sharpening stones also vary according to their composition and degree of coarseness. The Arkansas stone is a natural mineral stone and is hard with a fine abrasiveness (Fig. 13-34, right). The India stone is artificially made and is usually coarser (Fig. 13-34, left). The mounted stones are made of artificial substances and are generally fairly coarse. If the instrument is quite dull, a coarser stone should be used, but the less abrasive Arkansas stone is preferred for creating a fine cutting edge on an instrument that is only slightly dull.

The cutting edge of an instrument is formed

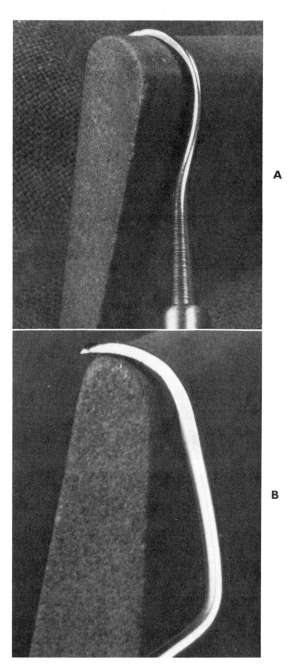

FIGURE 13-32. A, The larger rounded end of a tapered India stone is used to sharpen a universal curet. **B,** The smaller rounded end of a tapered India stone is used to sharpen a small Gracey curet.

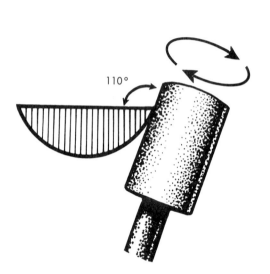

FIGURE 13-33. A mounted stone used to sharpen the blade of a curet on its lateral surface. Note the 110-degree angle between the stone and the face of the instrument.

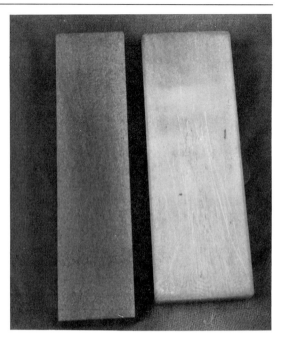

FIGURE 13-34. Flat India stone on the left. Flat Arkansas stone on the right.

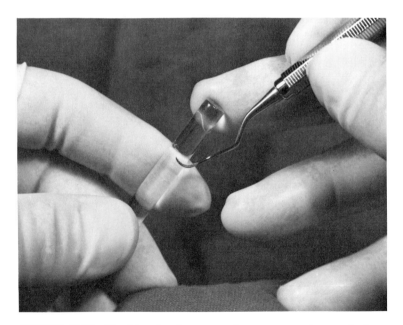

FIGURE 13-35. Checking the sharpness of a curet on a plastic cylinder.

by the meeting of two surfaces of the blade. A sharp edge is fine, smooth, and linear because it has length but no thickness. A dull edge is blunt and rounded and has thickness. Instruments can be checked for sharpness by using a magnifying glass and a light source. If the instrument is dull, the cutting edge appears as a shiny surface that reflects the light. A sharp instrument has a cutting edge that appears as a fine line that does not reflect the light. Sharpness may also be checked by applying the cutting edge to a plastic surface to see if it grips the surface with light pressure at the proper angle (Fig. 13-35).

Basic principles of instrument sharpening

1. Instruments should be sharpened at the first sign of dullness.
2. Working surface for instrument sharpening should be firm, stationary, and stable; an adequate light source must be available.
3. Instrument to be sharpened is held with a firm grip and a finger rest established if possible. If an unmounted stone is used, the stone should be stabilized with the opposite hand.
4. Stones of proper size and shape are used to avoid damaging the working end.
5. Surface of the sharpening stone should be lubricated with a thin layer of clean, light oil during sharpening unless sterile techniques prevent its use.
6. Before sharpening the instrument should be examined to determine the proper cutting edges, angles, and bevels. This is done to establish the proper angle of placement of the cutting edge on the surface of the stone.
7. The entire cutting edge is ground evenly to avoid creating a new bevel at the cutting edge.
8. Light but firm pressure is used; excessive pressure, which generates heat and reduces control, should be avoided.
9. The beveled edge of the instrument

blade is pulled against the sharpening stone. If the beveled edge is pulled away from the stone a "wire edge" is formed. This is a thin, unstable projection of metal from the blade, which will not remain sharp when used.
10. Check and test the sharpness of the instrument frequently. This is usually done after two strokes.

Sharpening procedures using a hard flat stone
Sickle scaler

Lateral surface.
1. Place the entire length of the cutting edge on the stone. The angle of the blade to the stone is determined by the lateral surface of the blade. Place it flat against the stone. This angle and position must be maintained during the entire sharpening process to provide for even sharpening (Fig. 13-36).
2. Use a short, slow, pull stroke as the instrument moves across the stone. Release pressure and slide the instrument back. Repeat the stroke as often as needed for ideal sharpness.
3. Turn the instrument and sharpen the other lateral surface in the identical fashion.
4. To sharpen the contra-angle sickle, use the same procedure as with the straight sickle, but use the side of the stone because of the curved shank.

Facial surface.
1. Place the entire facial surface flat against the side of the stone and maintain this stone-instrument angle during the process.
2. Use a short, slow, pull stroke.

Hoe scaler

1. Place the entire cutting edge of the instrument with the bevel flat against the stone (Fig. 13-37).
2. Sharpen the instrument with a pull

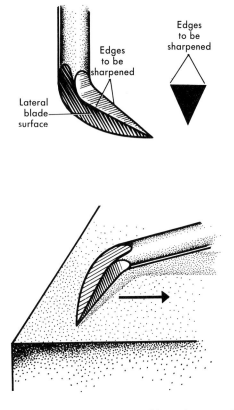

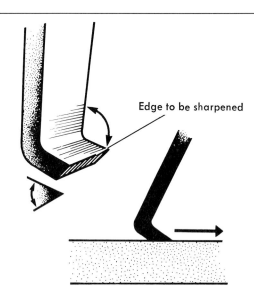

FIGURE 13-37. Sharpening a hoe scaler on a flat stone.

FIGURE 13-36. Sharpening a sickle scaler on a flat stone.

stroke across the stone, maintaining the proper angle.

3. Release pressure; slide the instrument back and repeat until sharp.

4. Round the sharp corners at either end of the cutting edge to prevent laceration of the gingiva and scratching the tooth surface when the instrument is used. To round the sharp corners, rub the surface of the stone over the corners with a gentle rolling motion.

Chisel scaler

The sharpening procedures for the chisel are similar to those for the hoe.

1. Place the beveled surface flat against the surface of the stone (Fig. 13-38).

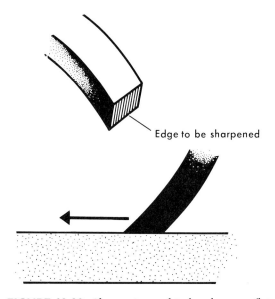

FIGURE 13-38. Sharpening a chisel scaler on a flat stone.

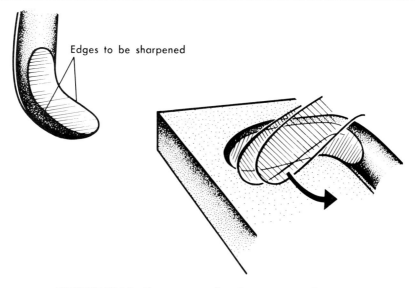

Edges to be sharpened

FIGURE 13-39. Sharpening a dental curette on a flat stone.

2. Push the instrument slowly forward across the stone, maintaining the stone-instrument angle. Remember that the stone should move against the cutting edge, not with it.

3. Round the corners by rubbing the stone over them with a gentle rolling motion.

Curet

1. Place the cutting edge on the stone at a 110-degree angle formed by the stone and the facial surface of the instrument (Fig. 13-39). Because the curet is a curved instrument, the entire cutting edge cannot be placed on the stone at one time; therefore sharpen the cutting edge with a series of strokes so that each portion of the cutting edge is sharpened.

2. Start by placing the cutting edge on the stone. As the instrument is pulled forward, turn it continuously along the cutting edge until the center of the rounded portion of the cutting edge is reached.

3. Release pressure and slide the instru-ment back. Repeat the stroke until the instrument is sharp.

4. Turn the instrument and sharpen the other side of the cutting edge with the same technique if the instrument is designed to be sharpened on both sides.

5. The curet can also be sharpened by holding the instrument firmly with one hand and moving the stone rather than the instrument against the blade with the opposite hand (Fig. 13-40, *B*). In either method the most important factor is that the angle between the stone and the face of the blade must be kept between 100 and 110 degrees if the cutting edge of the face to the lateral surface is to be maintained at 70 to 80 degrees (Fig. 13-40, *A* and *C*).

Care of stones

1. Stones should regularly be wiped with clean oil to remove the old oil and any particles that have accumulated after sharpening.

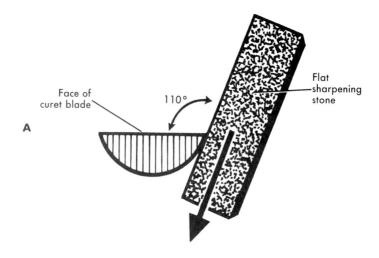

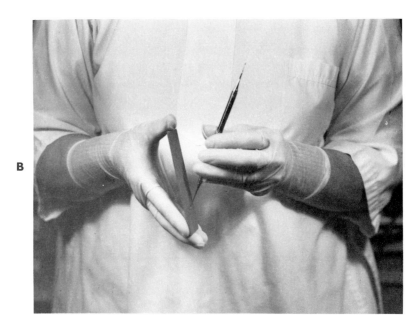

FIGURE 13-40. Sharpening a curet by moving the stone against the instrument blade. **A,** The 110-degree angle between the face of the blade and the stone. The movement of the stone is downward against the cutting edge. **B,** Hold flat stone with one hand and the instrument in the other hand. Press the elbows tightly against the body to add stability.

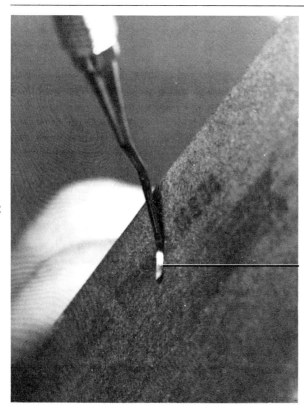

C

FIGURE 13-40, cont'd. C, Close view of the 110-degree angle desired between the blade face and the stone.

110°

2. When the surface of the stone has become blackened and clogged, the stone should be cleaned with gasoline or ammonia.
3. Stone should never be allowed to become dried; therefore it should be stored with a thin coat of light oil in a covered container.
4. Stone can be sterilized by autoclaving or boiling in a light oil. A contaminated stone can be a means for transfer of infectious bacterial agents.

SUGGESTED READINGS

Boundy SS, and Reynolds, NJ: Current concepts in dental hygiene, St. Louis, 1977, The CV Mosby Co, pp 101-114.

Carranza F: Glickman's clinical periodontology, ed 5, Philadelphia, 1979, WB Saunders Co.

Matsuishi A, and Pattison JB: Dental hygiene: the detection and removal of calculus, Reston, Va, 1973, Reston Publishing Co, Inc.

Pattison G, and Pattison AM: Periodontal instrumentation, a clinical manual, Reston, Va, 1979, Reston Publishing Co, Inc.

Wasserman B: Root scaling and planing, a fundamental therapy, 1986, Quintessence Publishing Co, Inc.

Wilkins EM: Clinical practice of the dental hygienist, ed. 4, Philadelphia, Lea & Febiger.

CHAPTER 14
Surgical Periodontal Procedures

Surgical periodontal procedures are employed as part of therapy to secure access and visibility for root surface debridement, to remove inflamed tissue, and to correct periodontal deformities that predispose the tissues to further periodontal disease and destruction. Gingival disease and early periodontitis with 3 to 4 mm probing depths are often treated with scaling and root planing (closed debridement) and effective plaque control. However, as periodontal pockets deepen through progressive destruction of the periodontal attachment tissues, plaque, calculus, and other tissue irritants accumulate in grooves, root concavities, and furcation areas, which are difficult to effectively instrument through closed debridement procedures. Therefore one of the indications for periodontal surgical procedures is to provide access for meticulous root preparation.

Another indication for periodontal surgery is to reduce the depths of gingival and periodontal pockets to create shallow sulci and physiological gingival contours that will permit adequate plaque control (Fig. 14-1). Deep pockets and rounded gingival contours contribute to the perpetuation of periodontitis by providing an ideal environment for the accumulation of plaque, which makes it difficult for patients to clean effectively. Pockets are reduced surgically through readaptation of the gingival wall of the pocket to the tooth, resection of the pocket wall, or regeneration of the periodontal tissues destroyed by periodontitis.

The last major reason for periodontal surgery is to correct mucogingival defects, which are areas with an inadequate zone of attached gingiva (Fig. 14-2). This correction is accomplished by creating or adding to the width of the attached gingiva. Adequate attached gingiva helps to prevent retraction of the gingiva by the muscles located in the lining mucosa and to create marginal gingiva that can withstand the frictional pressures of toothbrushing and food skirting off the teeth. Research studies have shown that attached gingiva is particularly important when restorations are placed subgingivally and in areas where the plaque control is less than adequate. However, when the plaque control is sufficient to maintain gingival health a zone of attached gingiva is no longer considered necessary to maintain periodontal health and stable attachment levels. Preliminary indications for periodontal surgery can be made at the time of the initial periodontal examination. However, the final decision to have periodontal surgery is generally made several weeks after the initial periodontal therapy has been completed. The reduction in the size of the gingival tissues following the meticulous removal of local irritating factors and the establishment of effective plaque control often eliminate the need for surgical procedures. Periodontal surgical procedures should not be performed until the patient has demonstrated a willingness and a reasonable ability to practice adequate plaque control. If the patient does not demonstrate cooperation with oral hygiene, it is better *not* to do surgery than to perform it and have a poor healing response. The level of the periodontal attachment and the depth of the healed gingival sulcus following periodontal surgery is directly related to the effectiveness of postsurgical plaque control.

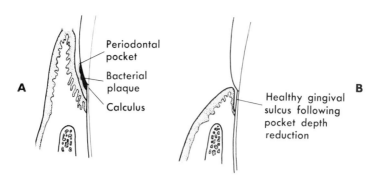

FIGURE 14-1. Pocket reduction. **A,** Typical periodontal pocket. Bacterial plaque in pocket is inaccessible to personal oral hygiene methods. **B,** Pocket has been reduced to a depth that will permit adequate plaque control and periodontal health.

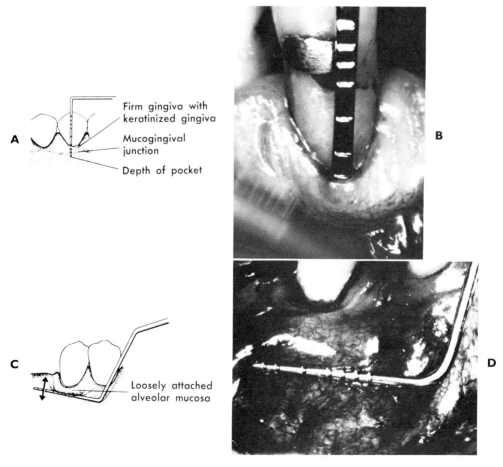

FIGURE 14-2. Mucogingival defects. **A,** Type I. The depth of the pocket is apical to the cementoenamel junction. Firm gingiva with keratinized epithelium is present, but it is not attached to the tooth. **B,** The blanching of the marginal gingiva over the probe to the mucogingival junction indicates that the sulcus depth extends to the mucogingival junction. **C,** Type II. The marginal gingiva is composed of loosely attached alveolar mucosa. **D,** Note the rolling of the alveolar mucosa in the marginal area.

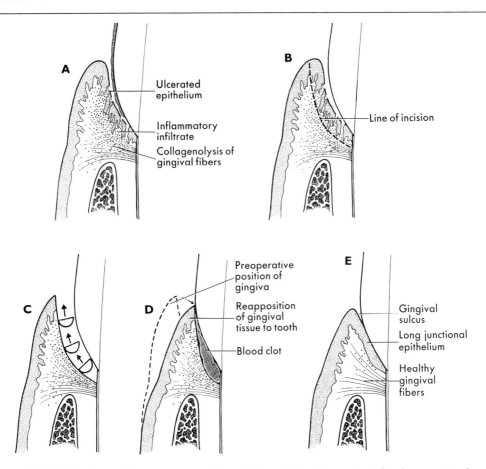

FIGURE 14-3. Gingival curettage procedure. **A**, Gingivitis. Note gingival enlargement, ulcerated epithelium, collagenolysis of the gingival fibers, and inflammatory infiltrate. **B**, Line of incision. Note that calculus has been removed from tooth. **C**, Multiple strokes with a curet are used to remove the crevicular epithelium and adjacent inflamed tissue. **D**, Reapposition of gingival tissue to the tooth and blood clot. **E**, Healed gingiva following the gingival curettage procedure. Note the shallow sulcus, long junctional epithelium, and healthy gingival fibers.

Following are the basic surgical procedures used to reduce pocket depths and create physiological gingival contours:

1. Gingival curettage
2. Gingivectomy
3. Periodontal flap procedures
4. Ostectomy and osteoplasty
5. Periodontal regeneration procedures

GINGIVAL CURETTAGE

Gingival curettage consists of removing the crevicular epithelium and adjacent chronically inflamed connective tissues in the soft tissue walls of pockets (Fig. 14-3, A). It is usually performed in conjunction with scaling and root planing of the tooth surfaces and is effective in reducing pocket depths by facilitating shrinkage of the gingival wall and/or the readaptation of the pocket wall to the tooth through a long junctional epithelium (Fig. 14-3, *E*). If the junctional epithelium is also removed, it creates an environment for the reduction of pocket depths by the new attachment of gingival fibers and epithelium on the root surface previously denuded by disease. While the latter is achieved in some cases, it should not be considered a routine, predictable procedure.

The principal clinical indications for this procedure are shallow (3 to 4 mm) pockets created by soft, boggy, edematous gingiva. The reduction of these pockets can be accomplished by eliminating the inflammation and edema in the gingiva and thereby allowing shrinkage of the pocket walls to take place. These types of pockets are frequently seen in gingivitis (Fig. 14-4) and early periodontitis (Figs. 11-19, *A* to *C*).

The procedure is performed as follows.

The patient's medical history is checked to make sure no contraindications to the use of local anesthetics or a surgical procedure exist.

Adequate anesthesia should be obtained in the area to be treated with local anesthetic. One quadrant of the mouth is usually treated at each visit.

All calculus and necrotic cementum should be removed from the root surface. This is frequently performed at a previous patient visit.

A sharp curet is inserted to the bottom of the pocket with the cutting edge directed toward the gingiva. While applying finger pressure on the external surface of the gingiva, the operator activates the curet with an outward and coronally directed stroke (Fig. 14-3, *C*). Several strokes with the curet are usually necessary to remove all the epithelium and the red, bead-like granulation tissue. The tissues may also be incised with a sharp blade and then removed with a curet.

Following the soft tissue curettage, the root surface should be checked with a fine explorer for smoothness. Any imperfections can be corrected at this time.

The instrumented pockets are then rinsed thoroughly with water, and depending on the extent of the tissue removal, a periodontal dressing may or may not be placed. The patient is advised to expect moderate discomfort. Warm water rinses are often recommended to ease the pain. Oral hygiene procedures should be performed by the patient in the other parts of the mouth as usual, with gentle brushing in the area of instrumentation or rinsing only in the areas covered by the periodontal dressing. An appointment should be made to see the patient in 5 to 7 days to remove the periodontal dressing and to check the healing.

Subsequent postsurgical appointments should be given at appropriate intervals until the tissue is completely healed. Further root planing, gingival curettage, and reinforcement of the patient's plaque control are often necessary during these visits.

The instruments used for this procedure include the following:

1. Mirror
2. Explorer
3. Medium size curet—for example, the McCall curets numbers 17s/18s or 13s/14s
4. Light finishing curets—for example, the Gracey curets

GINGIVECTOMY

The Gingivectomy procedure reduces pocket depths by surgically removing the soft tissue pocket wall (Fig. 14-5). The procedure is indicated for pockets that present the following clinical characteristics:

1. Deep gingival pockets formed by enlarged fibrotic tissue.
2. Deep suprabony periodontal pockets that have an adequate zone of attached gingiva. The latter must be wide enough to allow the entire beveled incision to remain in the gingiva.

Gingivectomy is contraindicated in the reduction of infrabony pockets and pockets ex-

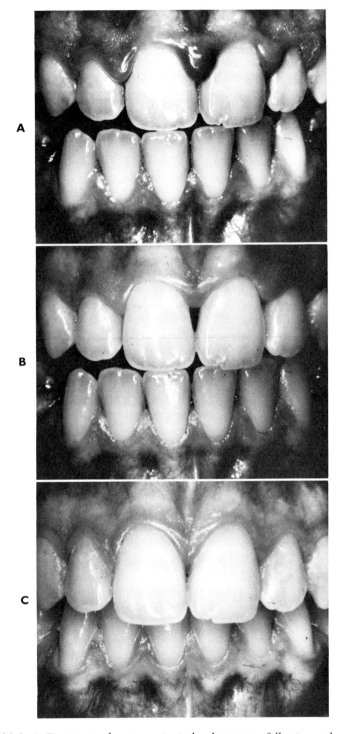

FIGURE 14-4. **A,** Persistent edematous gingival enlargement following orthodontic therapy in a 15-year-old girl. **B,** Same patient 1 month following plaque control instructions, scaling, and gingival curettage. Note blunted interdental gingiva during the early healing phase. **C,** Same patient 1 year following the gingival curettage procedure and periodontal maintenance therapy. Note the regeneration of the pyramidal shape of the interdental gingiva.

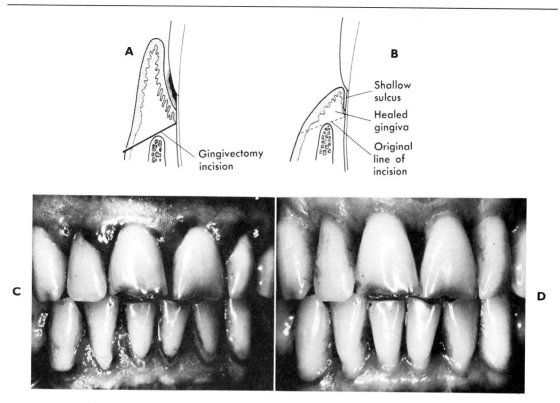

FIGURE 14-5. Pocket reduction by gingivectomy. **A,** Line of incision to remove pocket wall. **B,** Shallow sulcus following the healing. **C,** Moderate periodontitis in a 45-year-old patient. Suprabony pockets of 5 to 7 mm with adequate attached gingiva were noted. **D,** One year following the gingivectomy procedure and appropriate root preparation and oral hygiene instructions. Note more apical position of the marginal gingiva, which is tapered in contour and firm in texture.

tending to or beyond the mucogingival junction.

The procedure is performed in the following manner.

The patient's medical and dental histories are checked to make sure no contraindications to the use of local anesthetic or performing a surgical procedure exist.

Removal of most local irritating factors including calculus, overhanging margins of restorations, and caries and adequate plaque control must be achieved before doing any periodontal surgical procedure.

Adequate local anesthesia must be obtained.

One quadrant is usually treated at a time, and the appropriate nerve block and infiltration-type injections are administered. Supplemental injections into the interdental gingiva are sometimes added to reduce the bleeding during the procedure.

The depths of the pockets are marked with the pocket markers (Fig. 14-6, *A*) or a periodontal probe and recorded on the external surface of the gingiva with the bleeding points (Fig. 14-6, *B*).

The convex surface of a Kirkland number 15 or 16 knife or comparable gingivectomy knife is used to make the initial incision on the facial

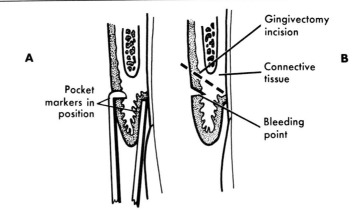

FIGURE 14-6. Recording the pocket depths on the external surface of the gingiva. **A,** Pocket markers in position. **B,** Line of incision is started just apical to the bleeding point marking the depth of the pocket.

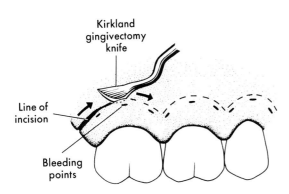

FIGURE 14-7. Initial gingivectomy incision with the Kirkland gingivectomy knife.

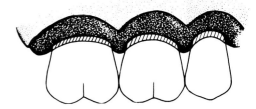

FIGURE 14-8. Gingivectomy completed. Gingival tissue has been removed, and the tooth surfaces are clean and smooth.

and lingual surfaces. The incision is started slightly apical to the bleeding point and is angled 45 degrees to the tooth (Figs. 14-6, *B,* and 14-7). A definite stroke should be used with either continuous or discontinuous scalloped incisions made directly to the tooth surface. This incision should remove the entire pocket wall, but a thin layer of connective tissue should be left covering the bone (Fig. 14-6, *B*). After the buccal and lingual incisions are completed, the interproximal incisions are made with a narrow, spear-shaped knife. The Orban numbers 1

and 2 gingivectomy knives or the Buck knife is recommended. The incision should extend horizontally underneath the interdental gingiva, separating it from the underlying connective tissue and completely eliminating the pocket.

When the tissue has been loosened with the initial incisions, a heavy scaler (CI ⅔) is used to remove the incised tissue.

Following the removal of the tissue, the curets are used to remove any remaining granulation tissue and to plane the root surfaces until they are smooth and hard (Fig. 14-8).

When the bleeding has stopped, a periodontal dressing is applied (Fig. 14-9).

Two basic types of periodontal dressings can be used: zinc oxide and eugenol dressings (example, Kirkland Periodontal Pack) or noneu-

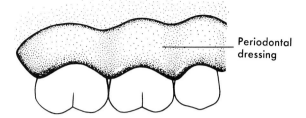

Periodontal dressing

FIGURE 14-9. Periodontal dressing applied to cover gingivectomy wound.

genol periodontal dressings (example, Coe-Pak).

The Kirkland Formula

Powder:

Zinc oxide	150.0 gm
Tannic acid	14.0 gm
Powdered rosin	198.0 gm

Liquid:

Lump rosin	70.0 gm
Sweet almond oil	29.5 ml
Eugenol	59.0 ml

Sig. Melt the lump rosin in the eugenol and add to the sweet almond oil. Mix powder to a thick puttylike consistency and apply. It is usually mixed before the surgical procedure has been performed. It can be stored (frozen) indefinitely.

The Coe-Pak Formula

Tube I:

Metallic oxides
Bithionol

Tube 2:

Nonionizing carboxylic acids
Chlorothymol

Sig. Mix about 1 to 2 inches of tube 1 to tube 2 until a firm consistency is reached, then apply. The material is quite sticky when first mixed but soon reaches a workable consistency. Petrolatum on the hands makes the material easier to handle. Since this dressing becomes hard within a few minutes, it should not be mixed until the surgical procedure is completed.

For placement either type of dressing is rolled between the palms of the hands to create a narrow cylinder. The cylinder is looped around the distal portion of the most terminal tooth in the group treated. It is then forced into the interdental spaces so that the buccal portion of the dressing is joined with the lingual side of the dressing. This provides the principal mechanism of dressing retention. The material should extend to cover the wound edges and be thick enough to give it strength. The surface should be smooth, and the edges should be accurately adapted to the underlying tissue.

The periodontal dressing is usually left in place for 1 week. At the time it is removed, the surgical wound is debrided and the healing is evaluated. If the operator believes the patient is comfortable and can perform adequate plaque control in the area, no further dressing is applied. However, if the surgical wound is still quite sensitive and only minimal epithelialization has occurred, a new dressing is applied for another 5 to 7 days.

The purpose of the periodontal dressing is to protect the surgical site from mechanical injury during the early healing phases. Periodontal surgical wounds have been shown to heal equally well with or without a periodontal dressing.

We recommend the application of a periodontal dressing as a protective measure until the patient can perform an acceptable level of oral hygiene in the surgical wound area. However, the use of antimicrobial mouthwashes following periodontal surgery has reduced the need for periodontal dressings.

The patient is given postoperative instructions (see the box on p. 215) and asked to return in 1 week.

The first postoperative visit consists of the following:

1. Removal of the periodontal dressing
2. Debridement of the treated area with gentle instrumentation and warm water
3. Recording of the healing progress in the patient's chart
4. Placement of a new periodontal dressing unless healing has progressed to the point that the patient can effectively use a toothbrush to clean the area

A subsequent surgical procedure can be performed at this time in an opposing quadrant if desired. It is suggested that the surgical appointments be arranged so that the patient has periodontal dressings on only one side of the mouth at a time. This enables the patient to masticate on the opposite side.

The patient should return again in 1 week.

At the second postsurgical visit the following are done:

1. Removal of the periodontal dressing if placed at the previous appointment
2. Debridement of the operated area, making sure that no food debris, plaque, or tooth deposits remain
3. Removal of any excess granulation tissue and root planing when needed
4. Polishing of the teeth
5. Review of plaque control instructions with an emphasis on cleaning the interproximal root surfaces, which are usually more exposed after surgery

The patient should return in 1 week. Another surgical procedure may be started at this appointment if needed. However, it is important to follow the healing progress weekly or at least biweekly until the tissues are pink, firm, and healthy. The new gingival sulci should be within 1 to 2 mm in depth. Failure to remove excess healing tissue or to insist on adequate plaque control can result in poor healing, return of pockets, and tooth sensitivity.

PERIODONTAL FLAP PROCEDURES

Currently flap procedures are the most common modes of periodontal surgical therapy. They are employed for four principal reasons: (1) to provide access to and visibility of the root surfaces, (2) to surgically reduce the depths of periodontal pockets, (3) to stimulate regeneration of lost periodontal attachment in periodontal pockets, and (4) to correct mucogingival defects. While certain procedures have been designed primarily to accomplish one purpose, in clinical use one procedure may accomplish several goals. For a detailed discussion of various periodontal flap procedures refer to the suggested readings at the end of this chapter.

Periodontal flap procedures are specifically used in the treatment of periodontal pockets that extend to or beyond the mucogingival junction and infrabony pockets. With these procedures the soft tissue portion of the pocket depth is reduced through one of two different techniques. In both methods the soft tissue pocket walls are detached from the teeth and bone, and the surgical area is thoroughly debrided, including root planing. With the replaced flap technique (modified Widman) the reflected gingival tissues are repositioned against the tooth at approximately the preoperative gingival height. This is done with the anticipation of reducing the probing depths through establishment of a long junctional epithelium or new epithelial and connective tissue attachments on the areas of the root that were exposed to the diseased pocket. With the apically positioned flap procedure the pocket depths are reduced by reapposing the reflected flap tissues at more apical positions on the teeth (Figs. 14-10 to 14-12). In this procedure the mode of pocket reduction is through physical movement of the gingival tissues in an apical direction, while in the replaced flap technique an attempt is made to reduce the pocket depths through a biological readaptation or re-

---

Postoperative instructions following periodontal surgery

The operation that has been performed for you on your gums will help you keep your teeth. Please read these instructions carefully. Following them will help make the surgery successful.

When the anesthesia wears off you may have slight discomfort. It is advisable to take a mild analgesic for this discomfort before the anesthesia wears off. Within the first hour following the appointment take two Tylenol tablets, then repeat the dosage every 4 hours as needed. If other medications have been prescribed, take them as directed.

You may have a periodontal dressing over your gums to protect them from irritation. The dressing helps prevent pain, aids healing, and enables you to carry on most of your usual activities in comfort. The dressing will harden in a few hours, after which it can withstand moderate forces of chewing without breaking off. It may take a short time to become accustomed to it. If a piece of the periodontal dressing breaks off or loosens and you are in pain or if a rough edge irritates your tongue or cheek, please call the office. The problem can be remedied by replacing the pack.

Follow a soft dietary regimen. Sticky, harsh, hard, brittle, crumbly, spicy, and highly seasoned foods should be avoided. The diet should be nutritive and bland, with a nonirritative consistency. It is advisable to do most of your chewing in an area of the mouth that does not have dressing.

Your usual oral hygiene measures should be maintained in the unoperated or previously treated areas of your mouth. In the area where the surgery was done, rinse with the prescribed mouthwash, but do not use a toothbrush.

There may be occasional blood stains in the saliva after the operation. This is not unusual and should stop in a few hours. If the bleeding persists, please call the office. Do not try to stop the bleeding by rinsing. Bleeding can be controlled by holding a piece of gauze with your thumb and index finger and applying it to both sides of the packing. Hold it firmly in place with pressure for 20 minutes. Do not remove it during this period to examine it. If after repeating this procedure the bleeding does not stop, contact the office or your dentist immediately.

Relax—healing after periodontal surgery is usually uneventful.

Special instructions:

_____

_____

_____

_____

_____

---

attachment of the pocket wall to the tooth. The advantages of periodontal flap procedures over the gingivectomy technique include the following:

1. Preservation of the pocket wall with keratinized epithelium. This is important if a mucogingival defect is present. If the pocket extends to or beyond the mucogingival junction, a gingivectomy incision to eliminate the pocket would remove all of the gingiva and leave only loose oral mucosa as marginal gingiva. The latter may not be conducive to long-range periodontal health.

2. Improvement of access to visualize and to treat intraosseous defects and furcation involvements.

3. Creation of a closed wound that can heal by primary rather than secondary intention.

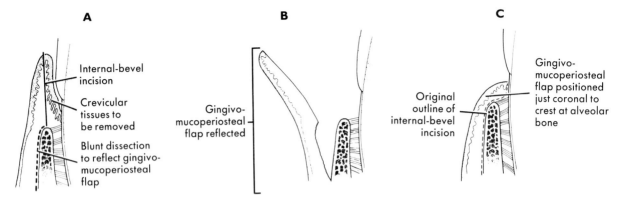

FIGURE 14-10. Apically positioned periodontal flap procedure. **A,** The internal-bevel incision removes the crevicular epithelium, the junctional epithelium, and the adjacent connective tissue. **B,** The gingivomucoperiosteal flap is reflected. **C,** The gingivomucoperiosteal flap is repositioned on the tooth just coronal to the crest of the alveolar bone. The pocket is eliminated by repositioning the pocket wall at a more apical level on the tooth.

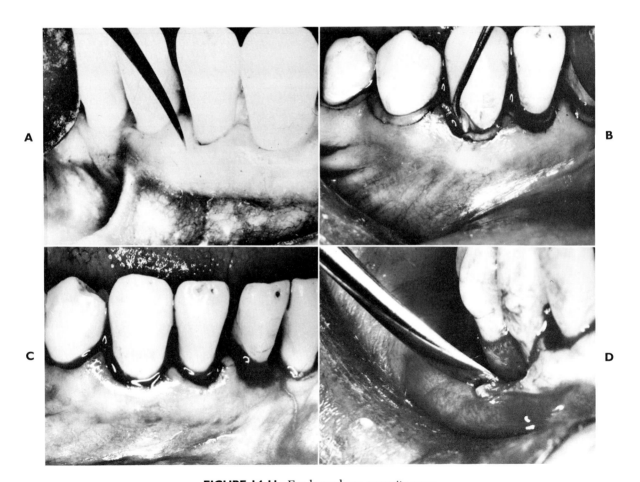

FIGURE 14-11. For legend see opposite page.

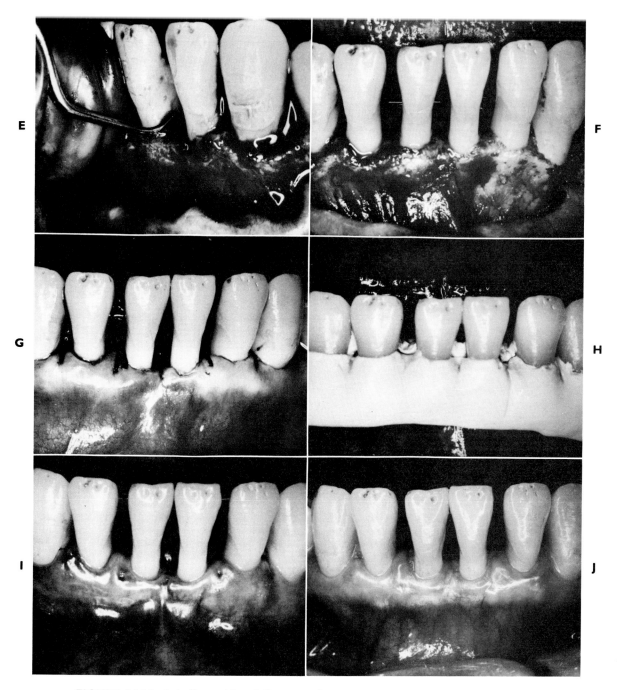

FIGURE 14-11. Apically positioned flap procedure. Patient is 45 years old and has periodontitis with 5 to 7 mm probing depths. **A,** Internal bevel incision with a 12B Bard-Parker blade. **B,** Removal of incised tissue with a curet. **C,** Gingival tissues following removal of incised crevicular tissues. **D,** Reflection of gingivomucoperiosteal flap with a periosteal elevator. **E,** Removal of granulation tissue and planing of the roots. **F,** Debridement and root planing complete. **G,** Apical positioning of flap at the level of the alveolar bone with interrupted sutures. **H,** Placement of periodontal pack. **I,** Healing after 1 week. **J,** Healing 6 months following surgery.

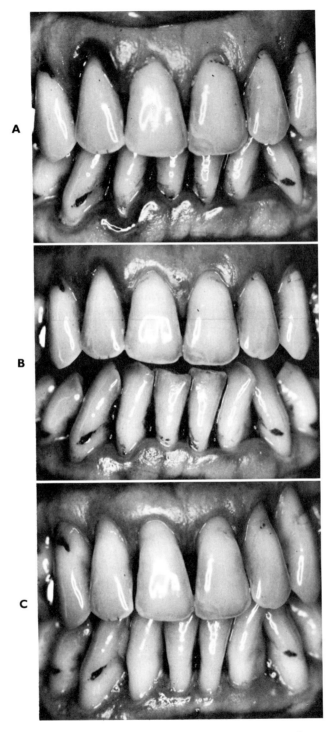

FIGURE 14-12. **A,** Periodontitis, chronic gingival inflammation, and 5 to 7 mm periodontal pockets in 45-year-old woman. **B,** Same patient following instructions in plaque control and scaling and root planing. **C,** Same patient following apically positioned periodontal flap procedures.

The primary disadvantage of these procedures is the increased injury to the radicular bone. Even if the periosteum is left on the bone when the flap is reflected, more surgical trauma to the bone is experienced than during a gingivectomy when no bone is exposed.

The apically positioned periodontal flap procedure is used when definitive pocket depth reduction is the primary goal (Fig. 14-12). The surgical procedure is done in the following way.

As mentioned in the gingivectomy section, it is important that successful initial preparation be done before a flap procedure. It is extremely difficult to accurately perform this technique when the tissues are red, friable, and edematous.

First, adequate anesthesia should be obtained in the area to be treated. A localized area involving four to six teeth is usually treated at one time. Larger or smaller areas may be done depending on the severity of the lesions involved and the skills of the operator.

The initial incision is called the internal bevel incision. It is begun at the crest of the marginal gingiva and terminates at the crest of the bone (Fig. 14-11, A). The incision extends circumferentially around the tooth and should excise the following:

1. Crevicular epithelium
2. Junctional epithelium
3. Portion of the inflamed connective tissue

The instrument of choice for this incision is usually a number 12B or 15C Bard-Parker blade. It must be extremely sharp to accurately perform a clean incision (Fig. 14-11, A).

A curet is used to remove the incised crevicular tissue and adjacent granulation tissue (Fig. 14-11, B and C).

The gingiva and the alveolar mucosa are then detached from the underlying bone with a periosteal elevator. The instrument is inserted between the gingiva and the tooth, and the flap is reflected by blunt dissection (Fig. 14-10, B, 14-11, D).

Vertical incisions at each end of the operated area are sometimes necessary to facilitate the flap reflection. However, they should be avoided if possible because they are a frequent source of postoperative discomfort. To minimize the surgical trauma to the bone, some periodontists recommend that only a partial thickness flap be reflected, leaving some connective tissue covering the bone.

The remaining granulation tissue is now removed with curets, and the roots of the teeth are planed until clean, smooth, and hard (Fig. 14-11, E and F). If osseous contours must be altered, they should be done at this time. (For details of this procedure see the following discussion of ostectomy and osteoplasty.)

Following the complete debridement of the area and the management of any osseous corrections, the flaps are repositioned around the teeth to just cover the crest of the bone (Fig. 14-10, C and 14-11, G). To maximize the width of the new attached gingiva, it is sometimes recommended that the gingiva be repositioned slightly apical to the crest of the bone.

In either case the tissues are held in position with interproximal interrupted sutures (Fig. 14-11, G). If a gingivectomy has been done on one side of the tooth and a flap on the other, a suspensory-type suturing technique is recommended.

When the bleeding has stopped, a periodontal dressing is placed (Fig. 14-11, H), and the patient is given postoperative instructions (see the box on p. 215). If the gingival tissues have been well readapted to the teeth with sutures, the periodontal dressing is often omitted. The use of antimicrobial mouthrinses reduces the need for more painful mechanical plaque control during the early healing period. The patient should return in 1 week (Fig. 14-11, I).

The first postoperative visit should include the following:

1. Removing the periodontal dressing and the sutures
2. Debriding the area
3. Recording the healing progress in the patient's chart
4. Placing a new periodontal dressing if the

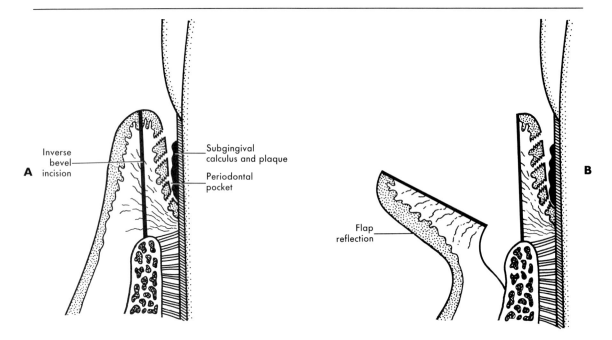

Inverse bevel incision

A

Subgingival calculus and plaque

Periodontal pocket

B

Flap reflection

tissues appear to be too tender to withstand the forces of toothbrushing

5. Making a new appointment for the patient in 1 week

The second postoperative visit should include the following:

1. Removing the periodontal dressing
2. Debriding the area and polishing the teeth
3. Recording the healing progress in the patient's chart
4. Reviewing the patient's oral hygiene procedures with particular emphasis on cleaning the interproximal root surfaces
5. Performing another surgical procedure if the tissues in the previously treated area are relatively comfortable

It is essential to observe the healing progress and the patient's plaque control weekly until the tissues are pink, firm, and healthy, with minimal sulcus depth.

The replaced periodontal flap procedure, also called the modified Widman flap procedure (Fig. 14-13), is used most frequently when the principal aim of the surgery is to reduce the pocket depths through readaptation

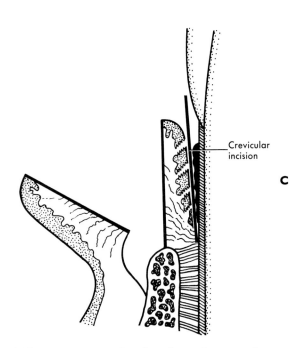

Crevicular incision

C

FIGURE 14-13. Modified Widman flap procedure. **A,** Inverse bevel incision. **B,** Reflection of gingivomucoperiosteal flap to expose crestal alveolar bone. **C,** Crevicular incision.

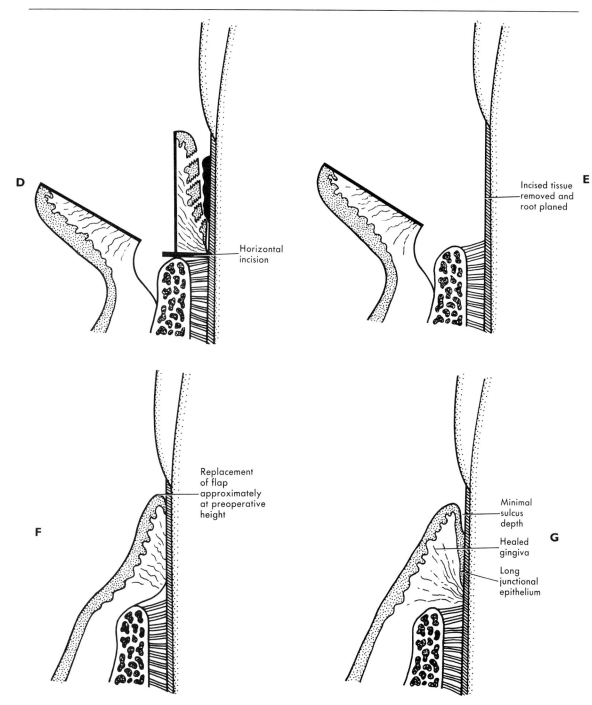

FIGURE 14-13, cont'd. D, Horizontal incision. **E,** Incised tissue removed and root planing complete. **F,** Replacement of flap at approximately preoperative height. **G,** Healed tissues showing pocket reduction through the formation of a long junctional epithelium and tissue shrinkage.

or regeneration and reattachment of periodontal tissues. With this technique the internal beveled incision is similar to that described in Fig. 14-10, *A*; however, the mucoperiosteal flap is not reflected from the bone as extensively, and following debridement of the surgical area and root planing of the teeth the flap is reapposed to the tooth and sutured at approximately the preoperative gingival height (Fig. 14-13, *F*). In addition to minimizing postoperative root exposure the advantage of this procedure is that it provides maximal readaptation of the periodontal tissues to the root surface to stimulate regeneration and reattachment. This flap technique also facilitates wound closure, which provides maximal postoperative coverage of the bone or grafting materials that are sometimes used to aid in the stimulation of tissue regeneration. A periodontal dressing may or may not be placed following the surgical procedure, and the postoperative course is similar to that described for the apically positioned flap technique.

OSTECTOMY AND OSTEOPLASTY

The ostectomy and osteoplasty surgical procedures are used to reduce the bony walls of infrabony pockets and to reshape abnormal alveolar bone contours that cause unphysiological gingival anatomy. In general the contours of the gingiva reflect the architecture of the underlying bone.

The term *ostectomy* refers to the process of removing alveolar bone that is directly attached to the tooth via the periodontal ligament-supporting bone (Fig. 14-14).

The term *osteoplasty* refers to the process of recontouring alveolar bone that is not directly supporting the tooth (Fig. 14-15).

Both of these procedures are done in conjunction with the periodontal flap procedure, which provides the necessary access to facilitate the instrumentation and the desirable coverage for the bone during the healing process. All of the details regarding initial preparation, surgical instrumentation, and postoperative

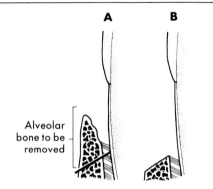

FIGURE 14-14. Ostectomy. Removal of alveolar bone directly attached to the tooth via the periodontal ligament-supporting bone. **A,** Alveolar bone to be removed. **B,** Bone contour resulting after ostectomy.

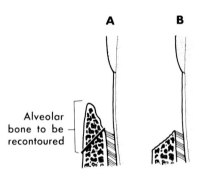

FIGURE 14-15. Osteoplasty. Recontouring of alveolar bone that is not directly supporting the tooth. **A,** Alveolar bone to be recontoured. **B,** Bone contour resulting after osteoplasty.

care described with the periodontal flap procedure apply to these techniques as well.

The infrabony pockets and other abnormal bone contours that are often treated with ostectomy and osteoplasty are as follows:
1. One-walled infrabony pockets (Fig. 14-16, *A*)
2. Two-walled infrabony pockets (Fig. 14-16, *B*)
3. Interdental osseous craters (Fig. 14-17)
4. Broad three-walled infrabony pockets (Fig. 14-16, *C*)

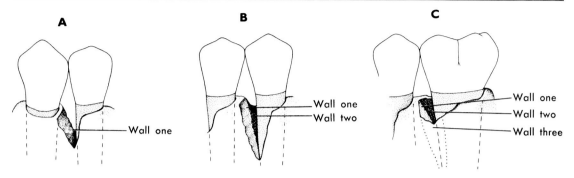

FIGURE 14-16. Infrabony periodontal pockets and abnormal bone contours. **A,** One-walled infrabony pocket. Only proximal wall of bone present. **B,** Two-walled infrabony pocket. Proximal and lingual walls of bone present. **C,** Three-walled infrabony pocket. Proximal, lingual, and buccal walls of bone present.

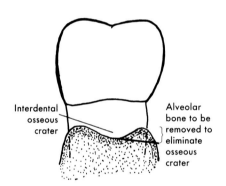

FIGURE 14-17. Interdental osseous crater.

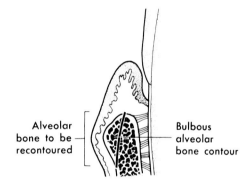

FIGURE 14-18. Bulbous alveolar bone contour.

5. Reversed alveolar bone architecture
6. Bulbous facial and lingual bone contours (Fig. 14-18)

The number of walls mentioned in describing the infrabony pocket refers to the number of walls of bone that are forming the osseous defect.

One-walled infrabony pockets can occur on the facial and lingual surfaces of teeth or on the proximal surfaces. The latter are also referred to as hemisepta. Both lesions are treated by removing the bone that is forming the pocket and sloping the remaining bone to establish tapering contours.

Two-walled infrabony pockets are also treated by removing the walls of bone that are forming the pocket and tapering the remaining supporting bone. Some two-walled defects are treated without removing bone in anticipation of periodontal regeneration to eliminate the defect. However, it is not considered to be a predictable procedure.

The interdental osseous crater is usually treated by removing either the buccal or the lingual peak of bone (Fig. 14-17). It is not usually necessary to remove both buccal and lingual peaks.

The broad three-walled infrabony pocket is usually treated by removing all three of the walls of bone that are forming the pocket and contouring the remaining bone. The narrow three-walled infrabony pocket can often be eliminated by the regeneration of destroyed periodontal ligament, alveolar bone, and cementum.

In reversed alveolar bone architecture the crest of the interdental bone septum is apical to the height of the adjacent buccal or lingual radicular bone. Bone contours of this type predispose to interproximal pockets. The bone architecture can be changed to be more physiological by reducing the heights of the adjacent buccal and lingual radicular bone to be just apical to the crest of the interdental bone septum.

The bulbous buccal and lingual bone contours are reduced by osteoplasty to create thin tapering contours (Fig. 14-18). This procedure aids in creating gingival contours that are more amenable to effective plaque control.

Following are the instruments used to remove bone in these procedures:

1. Hand chisels
2. High-speed coarse diamond stones or carbide burs with copious amounts of spraying water
3. Low-speed bone burs with copious amounts of spraying water
4. Small ronguers

PERIODONTAL REGENERATION PROCEDURES

Periodontal regeneration or new attachment procedures are also used in the treatment of infrabony pockets. With these techniques the infrabony pocket is eliminated by the regeneration of lost alveolar bone, periodontal ligament, and cementum rather than by removing the bone that is creating the defect (Fig. 14-19). Periodontal regeneration procedures can be used alone or in conjunction with ostectomy and osteoplasty. The narrow three-walled infrabony pocket lends itself best to these procedures. However, combination infrabony defects exist that only have one wall of bone at the crest of the pocket but have two and three walls of bone in the deeper portions. This type

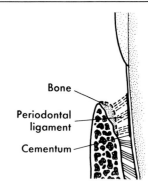

FIGURE 14-19. Regeneration of periodontal tissues: alveolar bone, periodontal ligament, and cementum destroyed by periodontitis.

of defect may be treated by removal of the superficial one- and two-walled portions of the pocket and then planing for regeneration of the periodontium in the deep three-walled portion of the pocket.

A detailed discussion of the periodontal regeneration procedures is beyond the scope of this book; however, currently the following basic procedures are being used:

A. Flap access and debridement
   1. Reflection of a gingivomucoperiosteal flap
   2. Surgical removal of the crevicular and junctional epitheliums and debridement of all granulation tissue
   3. Scaling and root planing of the teeth
   4. Accurate closure of the flaps with interrupted sutures and placement of a periodontal dressing
B. Epithelial exclusion techniques
   The flap access and debridement procedure is done as described above, but before replacing the flap a barrier material is placed over the osseous defect. This material retards the downgrowth of the epithelium and provides more time for the periodontal ligament and gingival fibers to attach to the tooth. Early reports of this technique are encouraging, but more research is needed to determine its predictability.
C. Grafting procedures
   In addition to the flap access and debridement procedure described above various materials are

placed in osseous defects prior to replacing the flap to facilitate regeneration of the destroyed tissues. Examples of materials that have been or are currently being used are:

1. Osseous graft materials
   a. Autografts (from same individual)
      (1) Cortical bone particles
      (2) Intraoral cancellous bone and marrow
      (3) Iliac crest bone marrow
   b. Allografts (from same species but different individual)
      (1) Frozen iliac marrow
      (2) Freeze-dried bone
      (3) Decalcified freeze-dried bone
2. Nonosseous graft materials
   a. Calcium phosphate ceramics
      (1) Tricalcium phosphate
      (2) Hydroxyapatite
      (3) Replamineform hydroxyapatite
   b. Cartilage
   c. Cementum
   d. Chondroitin sulfate
   e. Collagen
   f. Dentin
   g. Dura
   h. Gelfoam
   i. Methacrylate
   j. Plaster of paris
   k. Sclera

CORRECTION OF MUCOGINGIVAL DEFECTS

The surgical management of mucogingival problems depends on the type of defect present.

Type I mucogingival defects are characterized by pockets that extend apically to or beyond the mucogingival junction and a soft tissue wall of the pocket that is firm and covered with keratinized epithelium (Fig. 14-20, A). If deep periodontal pockets are complicated by type I mucogingival defects, the treatment of choice for pocket reduction is the apically positioned flap (Figs. 14-10 and 14-20).

Type II mucogingival defects are characterized by alveolar mucosa that acts as marginal gingiva with no zone of attached gingiva (Fig. 14-21, A). In this situation movement of the al-

veolar mucosa exerts tension on the marginal tissue, and the loose, friable alveolar mucosa is not able to withstand the forces of toothbrushing and food skirting off the teeth. This type of defect is often complicated by having a frenum or muscle attach into the marginal tissue.

The treatment of this defect usually involves transferring masticatory mucosa from some other location in the mouth to the involved area. Following are procedures commonly employed for this purpose:

1. Lateral sliding pedicle flap
2. Double-papillae flap
3. Free autogenous soft tissue graft

For the lateral sliding pedicle graft firm gingiva with keratinized epithelium is transferred from one tooth to an adjacent tooth (Figs. 9-13 and 9-14). This graft is indicated when an adequate donor site exists and when the objective is to cover a denuded root surface. It is contraindicated if the gingival tissues on adjacent teeth are thin and the teeth are prominently positioned, predisposing to bone dehiscences and fenestrations (Fig. 1-13). If the surgical procedure uncovers bone anatomy of this type, there is risk of causing recession in the donor site.

The double-papillae flap can be used when minimal donor attached gingiva on the adjacent teeth is found. In this procedure the interdental gingiva from the mesial and distal aspects of the tooth with a mucogingival defect are reflected and drawn together over the facial aspect of the involved tooth (Fig. 9-15). One of the principal advantages of this technique is the reduction in surgical trauma to the radicular bone under the donor tissue in the lateral sliding pedicle flap.

The free autogenous soft tissue graft is used extensively to restore gingiva to areas of type II mucogingival defects. This graft includes completely detaching masticatory mucosa in one part of the mouth and transferring it to the location of the mucogingival involvement (Fig. 9-16). The most common donor site is the palatal gingiva adjacent to the maxillary molars.

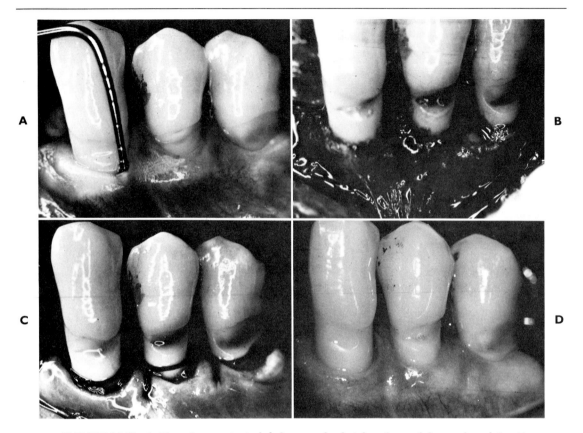

FIGURE 14-20. A, Type I mucogingival defects on the facial surfaces of the teeth and 5 to 7 mm interproximal pockets in 41-year-old woman. **B,** Reflection of a split-thickness gingivomucosal flap to provide access for debridement, root planing, and osseous recontouring. **C,** Apical positioning of the flap at the crest of the alveolar bone. **D,** One year following the surgical procedure. Note the elimination of the interproximal pockets and the increased zone of attached gingiva.

However, edentulous areas may also provide good, firm tissue suitable for grafting. This procedure is indicated when no attached gingiva on adjacent teeth is found and when the principal objective is to obtain an adequate zone of attached gingiva at the level of the bone (Fig. 14-21). It is not as effective as the lateral sliding pedicle flap in restoring gingiva to denuded root surfaces. However, it is considerably less traumatic to the radicular bone on adjacent teeth because the bone is covered with the graft during the healing process.

For more details on the management of the grafting procedure consult Chapter 9 or a more advanced textbook on periodontology.

TREATMENT OF TOOTH SENSITIVITY

An increase in tooth sensitivity to thermal changes is a common occurrence immediately following periodontal treatment. It is a particularly annoying complication, but usually of short duration. The hypersensitivity is most often related to a transient pulpal hyperemia resulting from the scaling and root planing or the removal or shrinkage of gingival tissues that provide a protective covering for the roots. The

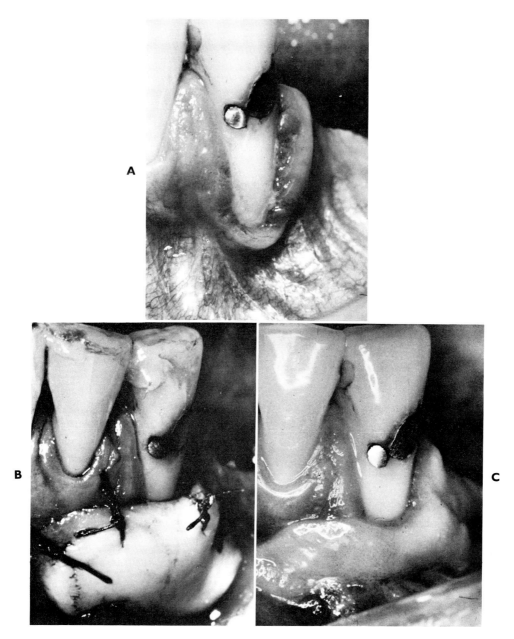

FIGURE 14-21. **A,** Type II mucogingival defect and gingival recession on tooth 22 of a 55-year-old woman. Note chronically inflamed, rolled, and friable gingiva. **B,** Free autogenous soft tissue graft from the palate is adapted to the tooth and sutured in place. **C,** One year after the surgical procedure. Note the wide zone of firm gingival tissue.

transfer of the stimulus on the surface of the dentin to the nerve endings in the pulp of the tooth is thought to occur through the odontoplastic process or by a hydrodynamic mechanism in which the fluid in the dentinal tubules is displaced. The burnishing of densensitizing agents onto the root surface is done to obturate the dentinal tubules and is thought to be effective because it interrupts the hydrodynamic mechanism of pain production. Severe isolated sensitivity may also be related to the exposure of a lateral pulp canal.

The severity and incidence of tooth sensitivity following periodontal therapy are directly related to the effectiveness of the patient's oral hygiene. It cannot be overemphasized that immaculate control of dental plaque following periodontal surgery is essential for the prevention of tooth hypersensitivity. If the microorganisms are allowed to accumulate regularly on the freshly scaled open dentinal tubules, the nerve endings will be continually irritated and sensitive.

The following precautions are helpful in the prevention of tooth hypersensitivity.

1. Meticulous plaque control before and after periodontal surgery
2. Periodontal dressing on the treated teeth until the gingival tissues have healed sufficiently to allow toothbrushing
3. Temporary restorations for carious lesions before the periodontal surgery

The treatment of hypersensitivity should always begin by perfecting the plaque control and by giving the pulp several weeks to adjust to the root instrumentation and the increased root exposure. However, if the tooth sensitivity persists, several office and home treatments are available. The basic mechanisms for the effectiveness of various desensitizing agents as explained by Pattison and Pattison are as follows.

1. Precipitation or denaturing of organic material at the exposed end of the odontoplastic process
2. Deposition of an inorganic salt at the exposed end of the dentinal tubules
3. Stimulation of secondary dentin formation within the pulp
4. Suppression of pulpal inflammation

The following are examples of various office or home treatments.

1. Burnishing of a sodium fluoride paste into the sensitive area on the root
2. Daily rinsing with a 0.5% stannous fluoride solution
3. Office and home application of a commercial densensitizing preparation such as Desensitizer (Lorvic Corp.)
4. Regular use of a desensitizing toothpaste such as Sensodyne, Thermodent, Promise, or Protect
5. Iontophoresis to deliver sodium fluoride into the root.

The procedures mentioned are also effective in the treatment of tooth sensitivity associated with idiopathic tooth erosion and gingival recession.

While the treatment of hypersensitivity is still partially empirical because the exact etiology and nature of the pain generation are not understood, it is amazing what meticulous plaque control will do for this annoying clinical problem.

SUGGESTED READINGS

Carranza F: Glickman's clinical periodontology, ed 5, Philadelphia, 1979, WB Saunders Co., Chapters 46 to 54.

Chaikin RW: Elements of surgical treatment in the delivery of periodontal therapy, Amador City, Calif, 1977, Quintessence Distributors.

Pattison G, and Pattison AM: Periodontal instrumentation—a clinical manual, Reston, Va, 1979, Reston Publishing Co, Inc.

Strahan JD, and Waite IM: Color atlas of periodontology, Chicago, 1979, Year Book Medical Publishers, Inc., Chapters 10 to 16.

Glossary

abscess localized inflammatory lesion consisting of purulent material (collection of pus) in a cavity; formed by the disintegration of tissues.

Actinobacillus actinomycetemcomitans (microaerophilic) small, gram-negative, nonmotile rods. Found in subgingival and marginal plaque and implicated as a major pathogen in localized juvenile periodontitis.

acute having a rapid onset, severe symptoms, and a short course; not chronic.

acute necrotizing ulcerative gingivitis (ANUG; Vincent's disease) inflammatory destructive disease of the gingiva characterized by necrosis and ulceration of the surface of the gingiva and punched-out, craterlike depressions at the crest of the gingiva; usually acute.

AIDS (acquired immune deficiency syndrome) a newly recognized disease syndrome characterized by breakdown of immunological function. Frequent concomitant pathological conditions include Kaposi's sarcoma and *Pneumocystis carinii* infection. The disease is found predominantly in the male homosexual population and among drug abusers. Viral etiology by the human immunodeficiency virus (HIV).

alveolar bone (alveolar process) part of the mandible and the maxillae that envelops the major part of the roots of erupted teeth, it develops with eruption of the teeth and is resorbed when the teeth are lost.

alveolar bone proper (cribriform plate) inner bony wall of the alveolus (tooth socket) comprising a relatively thin perforated plate adjacent to the root; consists of cancellous bone (with Sharpey's fibers forming bundle bone) except where the socket involves part of the cortical plate.

alveolar crest most coronal edge or portion of the alveolar bone, terminating at and parallel with the contours of the cementoenamel line.

alveolar mucosa that portion of the lining mucosa covering the alveolar process but excluding the masticating mucosa; it extends from the mucogingival line into the vestibule on the labiobuccal side or the floor of the mouth on the lingual side.

alveolectomy surgical excision of part of the alveolar process.

alveolus (alveolar socket) bony socket in the alveolar process in which the root of a tooth is held by the periodontal ligament.

anaerobe a microorganism that can exist in partial or complete absence of oxygen.

anaerobic environmental conditions which lack oxygen as a gaseous constituent. Also used in reference to microorganisms which grow under these conditions.

anomaly marked deviation from what is ordinary or normal.

antagonist tooth in the maxillary arch that occludes with a specific tooth on the mandibular dental arch or vice versa.

antibiotic substance produced by microorganisms which has the capacity to inhibit the growth of or kill other organisms.

antibody a specific substance, produced as a reaction to an antigen, that reacts specifically with the antigen in some observable way.

antigen a substance, usually protein, that elicits the formation of antibodies.

antimicrobial therapy the use of specific agents for the control or destruction of microorganisms either systemically or at a specific site.

atrophy decrease in size of a normally developed cell, tissue, organ, or part after having come to full functional maturity.

attached gingiva that portion of the masticatory mucosa firmly attached to the underlying teeth and alveolar process. It is bound coronally by the free gingival groove and apically by the mucogingival junction.

attachment apparatus   tissues consisting of the alveolar bone, cementum, and periodontal ligament, which support the teeth.

bacteremia   presence of bacteria in the blood.

bacterial plaque (microbial dental plaque)   complex, tenaciously attached soft deposit composed of a consistently organized structure of microorganisms, epithelial cells, leukocytes, and macrophages in an intermicrobial matrix and water.

Bacteroides   genus of obligate anaerobic, gram-negative bacteria. Several species have been implicated in human periodontal diseases.

  B. gingivalis   an anaerobic, gram-negative, non–spore-forming bacillus formally classified as *Bacteroides melaninogenicus* ssp. *asaccharolyticus*. *B. gingivalis* occurs primarily in the oral cavity and is associated with some forms of severe periodontal disease. It is a nonfermentative pigmented *Bacteroides* isolated principally from the gingival sulcus.

  B. intermedius   an anaerobic, gram-negative, non–spore-forming bacillus which was formally classified as *Bacteroides melaninogenicus* ssp. *intermedius*. *B. intermedius* is isolated from oral and other body sites. It is a common inhabitant of the gingival crevice and has been associated with infections of the head, neck, and pleura. There are two distinct DNA homology groups designated as *B. intermedius* I and II.

bifurcation   anatomic area where roots of a two-rooted tooth divide.

bifurcation invasion   extension of pulpitis or periodontitis into a bifurcation.

bite guard (night guard)   appliance worn on the teeth to evenly distribute occlusal forces over more teeth and to eliminate occlusal interferences.

bruxism   habitual grinding or clenching of the teeth, especially during sleep.

buccal mucosa   lining oral mucosa of the cheeks.

bulbous   bulb-shaped; swollen; terminating in an enlargement.

calculus   mineralized microbial plaque attached to and covering the enamel and/or root surfaces; two types—supragingival and subgingival—may be differentiated according to position during formation in relation to the gingival margin.

Capnocytophaga   a gram-negative, anaerobic, fusiform, rod-shaped organism found in dental plaque.

cardiopulmonary resuscitation   emergency manipulatory measures employed to maintain circulation of the blood and restore respiration, commonly referred to as CPR.

cementoenamel junction   boundary between the enamel and the cementum of the root.

cementum   mineralized connective tissue covering the external surface of the anatomical roots of teeth; the layer external to the dentin.

  acellular c.   cementum that does not contain cells; found mainly on the cervical two thirds of the root.

  cellular c.   cementum that contains cells; found mainly on the apical third of the root, in furcations, and as secondary cementum elsewhere.

chemotherapy   the prevention or treatment of a disease by chemical agents; often used in connection with antibiotics.

chisel   instrument designed for removal of interproximal supragingival calculus deposits, especially in the mandibular anterior area. It is used with a push motion.

chlorhexidine   a biguanide antiseptic agent used to prevent colonization of microorganisms on surfaces of skin, mucous membranes, and teeth.

chronic   persisting for a long time; showing little change or extremely slow progression over a long period; not acute.

citric acid   a tricarboxylic acid said to be useful in saturated solution (pH = 1) to detoxify (cleanse) diseased root surfaces and expose intrinsic collagen fibers in new attachment therapy.

cleft   fissure.

clenching   act of bringing the teeth together tightly and holding them or gnashing them together; gripping tightly; closing firmly.

clinical   pertaining to or founded on actual observation and treatment of patients.

col   depression between the facial and lingual peaks of the interdental gingiva.

collagen   fibrous insoluble protein found in the connective tissue including skin, bone, ligaments, and cartilage.

collagen fiber   type of connective tissue fiber. Gingival and periodontal ligament fibers are examples of collagen fibers.

contraindication   any symptom or circumstance indicating the inappropriateness of a form of treatment which is otherwise advisable.

crater   a saucer-shaped defect of soft tissue or bone, often seen interdentally.

crevicular epithelium (sulcular epithelium)   nonkeratinized, stratified squamous epithelial lining of the gingival sulcus, extending from the gingival margin to the junctional epithelium.

crevicular fluid (gingival fluid)   inflammatory product (derived mainly from plasma) secreted from gingival vessels exhibiting pathologically increased permeability; released via a gingival sulcus or pocket.

cribriform plate   name given to the alveolar bone proper because many small holes are present in which Sharpey's fibers and blood vessels are embedded.

curettage   surgical removal of the epithelial lining of soft tissue surfaces along the wall of a periodontal pocket.

curet   spoon-shaped instrument with two continuous cutting edges used to remove the soft tissue wall of a pocket and as a root planer.

cyst   sac or capsule containing a liquid or semisolid substance.

debridement   removal of lacerated, devitalized, or contaminated tissue.

degeneration   deterioration or impairment of an organ or part in structure of cells and the substances of which they are a part.

dehiscence   incomplete coverage by bone of a localized area of a root of a tooth, extending for a variable distance from the alveolar crest.

dental plaque   see *bacterial plaque.*

dentifrice   preparation composed of agents intended to clean and polish the teeth. Active ingredients to prevent caries and plaque accumulation as well as agents to desensitize the teeth may be included.

dentin   calcific tissue forming the body of a tooth, underlying the cementum and the enamel.

desensitization   abolition of sensitivity to a particular antigen.

desmosomes   structures that join epithelial cells together.

desquamation   exfoliation; the process of shedding surface epithelium.

desquamative gingivitis   uncommon gingivitis in which the oral gingival epithelium becomes extremely thin as a result of cellular desquamation and the gingiva is bright red and sharply demarcated from the tissue; many of the cases are considered to represent lichen planus or mucous membrane pemphigoid.

diabetes   general term referring to disorders characterized by excessive urine excretion, as in diabetes mellitus and diabetes insipidus.

diagnosis   art of identifying or recognizing a disease.

Dilantin   trademark for preparations of phenytoin. This drug is often associated with gingival hyperplasia.

disuse atrophy   decrease in the size of a normally developed organ or tissue as a result of its inactivity or diminished function.

dystrophy   disorder resulting from defective or faulty cellular nutrition.

-ectomy   excision (removal by cutting) of an organ or part.

edema   presence of abnormally large amounts of fluid in the intercellular tissue spaces of the body.

edematous   adjective used to describe tissues undergoing edema; pertaining to or characterized by edema.

embrasure   open space between the proximal surfaces of two teeth where they diverge bucally, labially, or lingually and occlusally from the areas of contact.

enamel   hard, calcified tissue that covers the dentin of the crown portion of a tooth.

enzymes   organic compounds that catalyze chemical reactions in living cells.

epithelial attachment   biological mechanism uniting epithelial cells of the junctional epithelium to the tooth surface.

epithelium (oral)   the tissue serving as the lining of

the intraoral surfaces. It extends into the gingival crevice and adheres to the tooth at the base of the crevice.

crevicular e.   the nonkeratinized epithelium of the gingival crevice.

junctional e.   a single or multiple layer of nonkeratinizing cells adhering to the tooth surface at the base of the gingival crevice. Also termed **epithelial attachment.**

sulcular E.   see **epithelium, crevicular.**

equilibration   reshaping, usually by grinding, of the occluding surfaces of the teeth to equalize occlusal stress.

erythema   redness of the skin caused by congestion of the capillaries.

etiological agent   causative agent.

etiology   science of causes or origins of any disease.

explorer   instrument used to locate subgingival deposits before scaling and to check the smoothness of the root after treatment.

exudate   material that has escaped from blood vessels and been deposited in tissues or on tissue surfaces, usually as a result of inflammation.

familial   occurring in or affecting members of the same family.

fenestration   incomplete coverage by bone of a root of a tooth, apical to the level of the intact alveolar bone crest.

fibroblast   a flat, elongated, spindle-shaped cell which synthesizes collagen and may be involved in collagen maturation and remodeling.

fibronectin   a glycoprotein that enhances cell adhension, wound healing, and hemostasis.

fibrosis   a fibrous change of the mucous membranes, especially the gingiva, as a result of chronic inflammation. Fibrotic gingiva may appear outwardly healthy, masking underlying disease.

file   wide, bulky instrument with multiple cutting edges used to remove calculus deposits and to smooth root areas in deep, narrow-mouthed pockets; also used to remove overhanging margins; used with a pull-type motion.

fistula   tract transmitting fluid or pus from an area of infection; commonly associated with abscesses.

flap (surgical)   surgical separation of one tissue from another.

free gingiva (marginal gingiva)   unattached, most coronal portion of the gingiva that encircles the tooth to form the gingival sulcus.

free gingival groove   a shallow V-shaped groove or indentation that approximates the free gingiva and runs parallel to the margin of the gingiva. It is seldom present.

freeze-drying   lyophilization. Isolation of a solid substance from a solution by freezing the solution and evaporating the ice under a vacuum.

fremitus   palpable or visible movement of a tooth when subjected to occlusal forces.

frenulum   a small **frenum** (see below)

abnormal f.   aberrant insertions of labial, buccal, or lingual frenula capable of retracting gingival margins, creating diastemas, and limiting lip and tongue movements.

labial f.   the fold of mucous membrane connecting the lip and the alveolar process in the midline of both the maxilla and mandible.

Lingual f.   the fold of mucous membrane connecting the tongue with the floor of the mouth and the mandibular alveolar process.

frenum   narrow band of soft tissue that attaches localized areas of the facial and lingual mucosa to the alveolar mucosa.

furcation   division of tooth roots at their point of junction with the root trunk.

gingiva   combination of epithelial and connective tissues that surrounds and is attached to the tooth and alveolar bone and extends to the mucogingival junction; on the palatal side it is a rim of tissue that merges with the masticatory mucosa of the hard palate.

gingival atrophy   loss of gingival tissue and crestal attachment apparatus, apparently noninflammatory, with concurrent apical shift of the gingival margin without pocketing.

gingival cleft   localized narrow area of gingival recession.

gingival fibromatosis (familial gingival hyperplasia)   rare and possibly hereditary disease associated with a fibrous thickened gingiva, not caused by chronic inflammation or by long-term phenytoin therapy.

gingival hyperplasia enlargement of the gingiva produced by an increase in the number of its elements.

gingival margin line or edge of gingival tissue representing the junction of the gingiva and sulcular epithelium; the most coronal line of gingival tissue.

gingival pocket (relative pocket, pseudopocket) pathologically altered gingival sulcus marked by an increase in the depth of the sulcus caused by an enlargement of the gingiva without destruction of the underlying periodontal tissues; a pocket that does not extend beyond the gingival tissues and is not associated with bone loss.

gingival recession loss of gingival tissue in an apical direction resulting in exposure of the root of the tooth either in the form of clefts or in a more generalized form; the latter form of gingival recession may be caused by inflammatory processes or chronic abrasive injury, and it may be related to the anatomical position of the teeth.

gingival sulcus (crevice) potential space surrounding the tooth that lies between the gingival crest and the bottom of the sulcus and is formed by the tooth on one side and the gingival tissue on the other; the shallow groove between the tooth and the most coronal part of the gingiva, extending from the bottom of the sulcus to the gingival margin.

gingivectomy surgical excision of gingival tissue to reduce the depth of the gingival or periodontal pockets.

gingivitis nonspecific term used to denote an inflammatory condition of the gingiva regardless of the etiology.

gingivoplasty surgical reshaping and recontouring of the gingiva to produce physiological contours.

glossitis inflammation of the tongue.

graft portion of tissue transposed from one location to another to correct a defect.

gram-negative (adjective) pertaining to microorganisms which do not retain gentian or crystal violet when decolorized by alcohol. They retain only the counterstain, resulting in a pink coloration.

gram-positive (adjective) pertaining to microorganisms that retain gentian or crystal violet stain, resulting in a blue color.

gram stain—positive/negative pertaining to histochemical reactions of bacterial cell walls.

granulation tissue healing tissue that consists of young fibroblasts, capillary buds, inflammatory cells, and edema (not to be confused with granulomatous tissue).

halitosis foul or unpleasant breath.

hemisection surgical separation of a multirooted tooth through the furcation area in such a way that a root or roots may be surgically removed along with the associated portion of the crown. The procedure is most frequently performed on lower molars but may be performed on any multirooted tooth.

hemorrhage bleeding; the escape of blood from a ruptured vessel.

herpes simplex virus that causes an acute infectious disease characterized by groups of watery blisters on the skin and mucous membranes.

histopathology the study of pathological changes within the structures of tissues at the magnification level of the light microscope.

hoe instrument used for planing and smoothing root surfaces and for removal of calculus remnants and softened cementum. A pull stroke is used.

hyper- over; excessive; above.

hyperkeratosis hypertrophy of the horny layer of the epithelium; thickening of the stratum corneum.

hypermineralization the presence of unusual amounts of mineral elements in a calcified tissue. Root surfaces sometimes become hypermineralized.

hyperplasia abnormal multiplication or increase in the number of normal cells in normal arrangement in a tissue.

hyperplastic pertaining to or characterized by hyperplasia.

hypersensitivity, dental the tendency of teeth to react painfully to stimuli such as thermal, mechanical, or chemical change.

hypertrophy 1. enlargement or overgrowth of an organ or part due to an increase in size of its constituent cells. 2. increase in the number or size of the cells of which a tissue is composed as the result of increase in function of that tissue. Not found in gingiva. See also *hyperplasia.*

hypo-   beneath; under; less than.

hypophosphatasia   an inborn error of metabolism characterized by reduced or absent alkaline phosphatase in the cells and serum, resulting in the defective formation of bone and cementum.

iatrogenic   abnormal mental or physical condition induced in a patient by the effects of treatment.

infection   abnormal or diseased state caused by invasion and multiplication of pathogenic microorganisms within the body.

infiltration   deposition or diffusion of substances not normal to a tissue.

inflammation   1. localized protective response elicited by injury or destruction of tissues, which serves to destroy, dilute, or wall off both the injurious agent and the injured tissue. 2. the cellular and vascular phenomenon that arises when a tissue is injured; the reaction of tissues to injury.

infra-   beneath; below; under.

infrabony pocket (intrabony pocket)   periodontal pocket in which the epithelial attachment is apical to the level of the adjacent alveolar bone.

interdental (interproximal) bone   portion of the alveolar process located between two adjacent erupted teeth of the same arch; consists of two cribriform plates and the supporting bone.

interdental col   concave interdental gingiva between the interdental papillae, apical to the contact area of adjacent teeth.

interdental gingiva   that portion of the gingiva located in the interproximal space created by adjacent teeth in contact.

interdental stimulation   repeated pressure applied to the crest of the interdental gingiva.

intermediate plexus   central zone of the periodontal ligament where the principal fibers from the cementum join with the principal fibers from the bone.

interproximal   between adjoining surfaces, as the space between adjacent teeth.

interproximal space   the space between adjacent teeth in a dental arch.

interradicular bone   portion of the alveolar process located between the roots of a multirooted tooth.

intrabony pocket   see *infrabony pocket*

irrigation   washing of a cavity or wound by a stream of water or other fluid.

irritant   local agent that produces a local inflammatory reaction.

-itis   inflammation.

junctional epithelium   epithelial collar that provides the epithelial attachment to the tooth surface, continuous with but structurally distinct from the sulcular epithelium.

juvenile periodontitis (periodontosis)   periodontal disease characterized by loss of attachment and destruction of bone adjacent to permanent first molars and/or incisors in children, adolescents, and young adults; other teeth may also be affected.

keratin   scleroprotein that is the principal constituent of epidermal tissue; main element of the stratum corneum layer of the epithelium.

keratinize   to become hard or horny.

laceration   wound produced by tearing or an irregular cut.

lamina dura   layer of compact bone forming the wall of a tooth alveolus; the alveolar bone. In a radiograph it appears as a thin radiopaque line separated from the tooth by the radiolucent image of the periodontal space.

lamina propria   the connective tissue layer lying deep to the epithelium which it supports; the comparable part of skin is known as the dermis. It varies in thickness.

lesion   broad term for any damage to a tissue.

leukocidin   substance produced by some bacteria which is toxic to leukocytes.

lichen planus   inflammatory mucocutaneous disorder characterized by discrete skin papules with a keratinized covering which often appears in the form of adherent scales. Oral lesions are common and are sometimes the only manifestation of the disease. Three types of oral lichen planus have been reported: (1) atrophic or annular form (most common), (2) hypertrophic or nodular form, and (3) ulcerative or erosive form.

lining mucosa type of nonkeratinized oral mucous membrane.

lymphocyte spherical cell of the lymphoid series, 7μ to 20μ in diameter with a large, round nucleus and scanty cytoplasm. It is the principal cell involved in the immune response. There are two major populations, T (or thymus-dependent) lymphocytes and B (or bursa-equivalent) lymphocytes. B lymphocytes may differentiate and become antibody-producing plasma cells, while T lymphocytes are involved in a variety of cell-mediated immune reactions.

lymphokines active mediators produced by lymphocytes (both T and B). They play a role in macrophage activation, lymphocyte transformation, and cell-mediated immunity.

macrophage large phagocytic cell, part of the reticuloendothelial system. Macrophages have a direct and important function in cellular-mediated immunity. They participate with T lymphocytes in aiding the response of B lymphocytes to many antigens.

maintenance the act or process of keeping something in an existing state.

    periodontal maintenance an extension of periodontal therapy. The continuing periodic assessment and prophylactic treatment of the periodontal structures that permit early detection and treatment of new or recurring abnormalities or disease.

malocclusion any deviation from normal occlusion caused by malposition of a tooth or teeth or an improper relationship of the jaws.

marginal gingiva see *free gingiva*.

mast cell a heparin-producing cell found in loose connective tissue along blood vessels; the name given to a basophil after it has left the bloodstream and entered the tissues.

masticatory mucosa portion of the oral mucosa consisting of the gingiva and the covering of the hard palate.

materia alba white curds of matter found on the teeth and composed of dead cells, food debris, and other components of the dental plaque.

melanin dark, sulfur-containing pigment.

microbiology the scientific study of microorganisms.

microbiota the microscopic living organisms of a region.

microorganism a bacterium or any organism of the animal or vegetable kingdom that is invisible to the naked eye.

migration, pathologic the movement of a tooth out of its natural position, usually as a result of periodontal disease.

mobility (of tooth) the degree of looseness of a tooth.

mouth breathing the process of breathing primarily through the oral cavity; frequently associated with gingival enlargements and inflammation.

mucobuccal fold (vestibular fornix) depression between the alveolar mucosa and the labial and buccal mucosa.

mucogingival term used to describe the *mucogingival junction* (see below) and its relationship to the attached gingiva, alveolar mucosa, frenula, muscle attachments, and the buccal and labial vestibule.

mucogingival junction junction of the attached gingiva and the alveolar mucosa.

mucosa mucous membrane.

mucous membrane membrane lining canals and cavities that communicate with the exterior of the body.

necrosis death of a cell or group of cells as the result of disease or injury.

neutrophil polymorphonuclear leukocyte; important defense cell against injury and infections, comprising 60% to 70% of the total white blood count. They engulf, kill, and digest microorganisms. Impairment of their functions appears to be related to the pathogenesis of juvenile periodontitis.

new attachment the reunion of connective tissue with a root surface that has been deprived of its periodontal ligament. This reunion occurs by the formation of a new cementum with inserting collagen fibers.

nidus 1. the point of origin or focus of a morbid process. 2. nucleus.

occlusal adjustment technical procedure of reshaping the teeth for the purpose of eliminating prematurities and interferences in the occlusion.

occlusal trauma (trauma from occlusion) damage in the periodontium caused by stress on the teeth produced directly or indirectly by teeth of the opposing jaw.

occlusion contacts that occur between the maxillary and mandibular teeth during mandibular movements and during certain static positions.

operculum hood or flap of mucosa over an unerupted or partially erupted tooth.

oral flora bacteria normally residing within the oral cavity.

oral hygiene (oral physiotherapy; patient's dental hygiene practices) removal of bacterial plaque with brushes, dental floss, and other special instruments; maintenance of oral cleanliness.

osseous bony; pertaining to bone.

ostectomy 1. excision of a bone or portion of a bone. 2. in periodontics the removal of some alveolar bone, thus changing the position of crestal bone on the tooth root. Ostectomy is done to reshape deformities caused by periodontitis in the marginal and interalveolar bone.

osteoblast a cell which arises from mesenchymal tissue and is associated with the production of bone.

osteoclast a large multinuclear cell associated with the absorption and the removal of bone.

osteocyte an osteoblast that has become embedded within the bone matrix.

osteoplasty reshaping of the alveolar process to achieve a more physiologic form without removal of alveolar (supporting) bone.

overhang excess of dental filling material extending beyond cavity margins.

papillary gingiva that portion of the marginal gingiva occupying the interproximal space.

pathogen any disease-producing microorganism or material.

pathogenesis the origin and development of disease.

pathology scientific study of the alterations or changes that cause or are caused by disease.

penicillin one of a group of natural or synthetic antibiotics originally obtained from cultures of the fungus *Penicillium*. It has a relatively broad spectrum of activity, inhibiting bacterial cell formation. Used chiefly in the treatment of gram-positive infections. Bactericidal in sufficiently high concentration.

percussion the art of striking a part with short, sharp blows as an aid in diagnosing conditions of the underlying parts by the sound obtained. Also useful in locating a tooth with an inflamed pulp through the pain response.

peri- a Latin prefix meaning around, surrounding.

periapical abscess localized suppurative inflammation of tissues around the apex of the root of a tooth.

pericoronitis acute inflammation of the gingiva surrounding a partially erupted tooth.

periodontal situated or occurring around a tooth; pertaining to the periodontium.

   p. abscess (lateral abscess) acute, inflammatory, destructive process in the periodontium resulting in a localized collection of pus; originates laterally to the root, usually emanating from a preexisting pocket; may become chronic with a draining tract.

   p. atrophy decrease in the size of the periodontium by the loss of cells and their products; an example is disuse atrophy.

   p. bony defects
      crater A wide-mouthed cup or bowl-shaped defect in the interalveolar bone with bone destruction nearly equal on the roots of the contiguous teeth. The side walls of the crater are formed by marginal bone on the vestibular and lingual surfaces, and these walls may be of unequal height.

      hemiseptum the remaining interdental bony septum where the mesial or distal part has been destroyed. A half septum remaining on one of two adjacent teeth.

   p. defects in marginal bone
      inconsistent margin vertical defects caused by uneven resorption of marginal bone. Also can be related to a supra- or infraerupted tooth or teeth.

   p. disease Those pathologic processes affecting the periodontium, most often gingivitis and periodontitis.

   p. dressing A surgical dressing applied over, and protecting, the surgical wound created by periodontal surgical procedures.

p. instrumentarium Instruments and supplies used in periodontal treatment.

p. interradicular defects

furca (furcal) invasion loss of bone in the furca of a multirooted tooth.

class I: minimal, but notable, loss of bone in a furca.

class II: a variable degree of bone destruction in a furca but not extending through the furcation to another tooth surface.

class III: bone resorption extending through the furca to another tooth surface.

p. intrabony defect a periodontal defect within the bone surrounded by one, two, or three bony walls or a combination thereof.

p. ligament the connective tissue structure that surrounds the tooth root and attaches it to the alveolus; the periodontal membrane.

p. membrane periodontal ligament. During eruption, this structure is membranous in nature, whereas, when the tooth is in function, the tissue assumes a more ligamentous form.

p. pocket a pathologic fissure bordered on one side by the tooth and on the opposite side by crevicular epithelium and limited at its apex by the junctional epithelium. It is an abnormal apical extension of the gingival crevice caused by migration of the junctional epithelium along the root as the periodontal ligament is detached by a disease process.

complex pocket a spiral type of periodontal pocket on more than one surface of the tooth but communicating with the gingival margin only along the surface at which it originates.

compound pocket a periodontal pocket on more than one tooth surface communicating with the gingival margin along each of the affected surfaces.

gingival pocket see *gingival pocket* above.

intrabony pocket a periodontal pocket that extends into an intrabony periodontal defect (see *periodontal bony defect* and *intrabony defect*.)

pseudopocket deepening of the gingival crevice resulting primarily from an increase in bulk of the gingiva without apical migration of the junctional epithelium or appreciable destruction of the underlying tissue. See *gingival pocket.*

simple pocket periodontal pocket on one tooth surface.

suprabony pocket periodontal pocket that has a base coronal to the alveolar bone.

p. probe a calibrated probe used to measure the depth and determine the configuration of a periodontal pocket and the condition of the crevicular epithelium.

p. probing (measurement of probing depth) insertion of a periodontal probe with gentle pressure between the tooth and the gingiva and measuring the distance of insertion.

p. space the space between the tooth root and alveolar bone containing the periodontal ligament.

p. traumatism pathosis induced by occlusal trauma.

periodontics that branch of dentistry that deals with the diagnosis and treatment of diseases and conditions of the supporting and surrounding tissues of the teeth or their implanted substitutes.

periodontist dental practicioner who by virtue of special knowledge and training in the field limits his or her practice or activities to periodontics.

periodontitis inflammation of the supporting tissues of the teeth. Usually a progressively destructive change leading to loss of bone and periodontal ligament. An extension of inflammation from gingiva into the adjacent bone and ligament.

adult p. periodontitis that usually has an onset after 35 years of age. Bone resorption progresses slowly and predominantly in the horizontal direction. Well-known local environmental factors are prominent, and peripheral blood-cell defects have not been found.

juvenile p. periodontitis that usually has its onset at puberty. It is characterized by vertical type bony defects on the first permanent molars; the incisors may also be affected. There is usually little or no clinical evidence of inflammation; there is a familial distribution, and the disease affects girls more often than boys. Patients studied have functional defects in either neutrophils or monocytes but not in both types.

necrotizing ulcerative gingivo-periodontitis periodontitis that follows long-term repeated episodes of acute necrotizing ulcerative gingivitis. The destruction causes predominantly interproximal crater formation in both soft tissue and bone. This form of periodontitis is also cyclic, and maintenance is difficult.

prepubertal periodontitis that starts soon after eruption of the primary teeth.

rapidly progressive periodontitis that usually begins between puberty and 35 years of age but may start much later. It may be associated with systemic disease, but it also affects otherwise healthy people. It may respond to rational therapy, or it may be refractory to all forms of therapy.

periodontium the tissues that invest and support the teeth—gingiva, alveolar mucosa, cementum, periodontal membrane, and the alveolar and supporting bone.

periodontology the scientific study of the periodontium in health and disease.

periosteum a specialized connective tissue covering all bones of the body and possessing bone-forming potential.

phase contrast microscopy method of microscopy that takes advantage of differences in light waves passing through transparent objects. The resulting differences are visualized as varying light intensities allowing for better differentiation of internal structures of the examined specimen.

phenytoin (Dilantin; diphenylhydantoin) anticonvulsant drug used in the control of epilepsy and other disorders and often associated with gingival hyperplasia.

physiological normal; not pathological.

plaque any organized mass, consisting mainly of microorganisms, that adheres to the tooth or occupies the gingival crevice. Besides microorganisms, plaque consists of an organic, polysaccharide-protein matrix, bacterial by-products, including enzymes, and inorganic components such as calcium and phosphorus.

predisposing factor factor that makes a condition more likely to occur.

pregnancy tumor pyogenic granuloma of the gingiva occurring during pregnancy.

preliminary treatment (periodontal maintenance,

prophylactic procedures for periodontal patients) procedures performed at intervals that assist the periodontal patient in maintaining dental health, including examination, evaluation of daily oral hygiene procedures and nutrition, scaling and root planing, and polishing the teeth.

primary occlusal trauma lesion that results when an excessive force is exerted on a tooth with normal bone support.

prognosis probable outcome of a disease.

proliferation reproduction or multiplication of similar forms.

prophylaxis, oral removal of plaque, calculus, and stains from the exposed and unexposed surfaces of the teeth by scaling and polishing as a preventive measure for the control of local irritational factors.

pseudopocket see *gingival pocket.*

purulent containing or consisting of pus.

pus thick fluid composed of viable and necrotic polymorphonuclear leukocytes; tissue breakdown products produced in infections from certain bacteria.

radiolucent permitting the passage of radiant energy; term used to refer to structures that appear dark in developed radiographic films.

radiopaque not permitting the passage of radiant energy; term used to refer to structures that appear light in developed radiographic films.

reattachment reunion of connective tissue with a root surface on which viable periodontal tissue is present; not to be confused with *new attachment* (see above).

recession location of marginal periodontal tissues apical to the cementoenamel junction.

  gingival r. location of the gingival margin apical to the cementoenamel junction.

  surgical r. location of the marginal tissues apical to the cementoenamel junction as a result of periodontal surgery.

regeneration natural replacement of a lost or injured organ or part.

resilient able to recover quickly and spring back to original form.

root planing definitive treatment procedure designed to remove cementum or surface dentin that is rough, impregnated with calculus, or contaminated with toxins or microorganisms.

root resorption loss or blunting of some portion of a root, sometimes idiopathic, but also associated with orthodontic tooth movement, inflammation, trauma, and neoplasia.

scaler instrument for removing calculus or other deposits from the surfaces of teeth.

scaling instrumentation of the crown and root surfaces of the teeth to remove plaque, calculus, and stains from these surfaces.
deep scaling subgingival scaling.

secondary occlusal trauma lesion that results when normal occlusal forces become excessive because of loss of periodontal support.

septicemia morbid condition caused by pathogenic bacteria and their associated poisons in the blood.

sextant one of the six relatively equal sections into which the dental arches can be divided.

Sharpey's fibers those portions of the principal fibers of the periodontal ligament that are embedded in either root cementum or alveolar bone proper.

specialized mucosa part of the oral mucous membrane; the dorsum of the tongue, which is modified for taste reception.

spirochetes (anaerobic) spiral-shaped, gram-negative bacteria characterized by flexible cell walls and internal flagella. Almost always associated with periodontal disease. Clinically significant genus: *Treponema* sp.

splint any apparatus, appliance, or device employed to prevent motion or displacement of fractured or movable parts.
dental splint an appliance designed to immobilize and stabilize mobile (loose) teeth.

stain pigmented substance, either on or within the tooth, that results in an abnormal discoloration.

Stillman's cleft V-shaped indentation extending from and into the gingival margin for varying distances.

stippling pitted, orange-peel appearance of healthy attached gingiva.

stomatitis inflammation of the oral mucosa.

subgingival area apical to the free gingival margin.

subgingival calculus calculus apical to the gingival margin.

substantivity the property of a substance to bind to either soft or hard tissues. In periodontics the term often refers to the binding characteristics of an antibiotic to the tooth or the gingiva.

succedaneous dentition the secondary or permanent set of teeth that replace primary or deciduous teeth.

succession sequential populational changes of the microbiota which accompany physiological changes in localized areas of the infected host.

sulcus bottom coronal termination of the junctional epithelium.

suppuration act of forming and discharging pus.

suprabony pocket periodontal pocket with the epithelial attachment located coronal to the alveolar crest.

supragingival area coronal to the free gingival margin.

surgery The branch of medical science concerned with the treatment of diseases or injuries by manual operation.
mucogingival s. plastic surgical procedures designed to correct defects in the morphology, position and/or amount of gingiva surrounding the teeth.
periodontal s. surgical procedure used to treat periodontal disease or to modify the morphologic status of the periodontium.
osseous s. periodontal surgery which deals with the modification of the bony support of the teeth. See *ostectomy, osteoplasty.*
reentry s. second stage procedure accomplished to improve or enhance results obtained from the initial operation.

temporomandibular joint (TMJ) joint formed by the condyles of the mandible and the mandibular fossa of the temporal bone.

tenacious holding fast; adhesive; sticky.

tetracycline antibiotic produced by certain strains of *Streptomyces.* Its administration during tooth formation may lead to enamel discoloration. Frequently used as adjunctive therapy in the management of juvenile periodontitis.

toothbrush trauma   Gingival recession or injury from incorrect brushing methods, usually with a stiff textured brush.

transeptal (fibers)   collagenous fibers that extend interproximally coronal to the interdental bony septa and are imbedded in the cementum of the adjacent teeth. Also spelled *transseptal*.

trauma   wound or injury.

trismus   difficulty in opening the mouth.

trifurcation   1. division into three branches. 2. area where the tooth divides into three or more distinct roots.

   trifurcation invasion   extension of periodontitis into a trifurcation area.

ulcer   local defect on the lining of a mucous mem-brane surface produced by sloughing of necrotic inflammatory tissue.

ulceration   formation of an ulcer.

ultrasonic scaler   instrument with a tip attached to a transducer through which high-frequency current causes ultrasonic vibrations, usually accompanied by a stream of water. These vibrations (approximately 25,000 Hz) produce a turbulence which removes adherent deposits from the teeth.

vesicle   circumscribed, elevated, fluid-containing lesion of the skin.

vestibular fornix   see *mucobuccal fold.*

SUGGESTED READINGS

Glossary of periodontic terms, J Periodontol, Supplement, November, 1986.

Index